I0437914

ALTERNATIVES

A Short Story and First-hand Anecdotes
Of Chiropractic Medicine
Story & Cummins

Written by
Robert T. Story, D.C.

Edited by
Marita R. Cummins

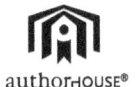

authorHOUSE®

AuthorHouse™
1663 Liberty Drive
Bloomington, IN 47403
www.authorhouse.com
Phone: 1-800-839-8640

First published by AuthorHouse 4/28/2009

ISBN: 978-1-4389-8174-1 (sc)

Printed in the United States of America
Bloomington, Indiana

This book is printed on acid-free paper.

ACKNOWLEDGEMENTS

It has been written and often repeated that no one writes a book alone. This book is no exception. I am indeed fortunate to have a lovely and talented cousin, Marita Cummins, to whom I am indebted for not only editing countless drafts but for lending her expertise and imagination in the development of various situations. Further, I am grateful for the knowledge obtained from such noted health care professionals as Jonathan Wright, M.D., Julian Whitaker, M.D., David Williams, D.C. and William Douglass, M.D. as well as the Health Sciences Institute and their informative articles and booklets. I also appreciate the wealth of information contained in Kevin Trudeau's three volumes of "Natural Cures They Don't Want You To Know About" which singularly launched me into the wonderful world of alternative health.

RTS

To lifelong learning students everywhere.

Learn all that you can,
Because life is the final exam.

Anon.

PART ONE

Part one is a fictional story. All names and events are fictional and any resemblance to actual names, places or events is purely coincidental.

Chapter 1

NANCY HOLT

The den is paneled with cherry wood. The focal point of the entire room though is a rather large and striking rustic stone fireplace with a mantel fashioned from railroad ties. On it rests an antique Seth Thomas clock which Nancy inherited from her parents and always seems to need winding. Bob inherited the winding detail and often wondered why an eight day clock needed winding every three days. Also on the mantel are two brass candlesticks and pictures of their lovely daughters, Meghan and Elizabeth. The functional aspect of the room, though, remains a pair of La-Z Boy gliders positioned to comfortably view a plasma television set. Nancy and Bob Holt spend many comfortable and relaxing hours, in this their favorite room, reading, viewing TV and just talking with one another. This night was such a time. With the galley in ship shape and their stereo softly playing Beethoven's 'Eroica' they were relaxing in their La-Z Boys reminiscing about their courtship days. They had met while in high school. He eyed her from a distance in the school cafeteria one day and was drawn immediately by her striking beauty. A friend later arranged an introduction – and the rest is history as they say. They reminisced about some of the special dates they had including parties, proms etc.

and even some of the pitfalls and heart aches they had both endured over the years. They always enjoyed one another's company and had their conversations in the den rather than the bedroom because about a year or so ago Bob contracted congestive heart disease which separated them into different bedrooms. With this disease congestion occurs in the lungs making breathing very difficult especially while lying down. Breathing becomes quite loud and very labored making it quite objectionable to others who might be sleeping in the same room. There are even times when breathing stops altogether for short periods. Doctors refer to this apnea as Cheyne-Stokes syndrome. So Nancy eventually took over the master suite while Bob settled into the guest room.

This night was no different as Nancy started through their nightly bedtime routine by shutting off lights and unplugging appliances not in use. She had a thing about unplugging appliances including the television even when the house was occupied.

"Hey, I'm still watching the news", cried Bob, as she flicked the television off.

"Oh, I thought you were going to bed too. When you do be sure to unplug it, please." Bob got up from his chair and kissed and hugged her goodnight. After embracing they looked at one another, grinned and almost simultaneously said "Don't forget to unplug the TV." Bob gave her a light spank on her rear end as she turned and headed down the hall to her room. Little did Bob realize that it would be the last time he saw her walk down that hall to her room.

At 11:00 o'clock when the news was over Bob shut the TV off and with a slight grin on his face remembered to also unplug it. He then checked to see that all doors and windows were closed and locked and that all lights were off before he went to his room. Before getting into his pajamas he went through his nightly hygienic routine in the full sized bathroom adjacent to the guestroom. And, as in the past, he vowed to get rid of the gaudy pink tile some day. They had bought this house eight years ago and every year he swore that he was going to rip that awful tile off the wall and floor and replace it with something more traditional. Maybe this year, he thought. When he crawled into bed and shut off the light he noticed that a light in Nancy's room was still on. She must be reading he reasoned but thought nothing of it as she was in the habit of doing that quite often. Not suspecting anything out of the ordinary he promptly fell off to sleep.

Later that night something caused Bob to stir and when he was fully awake he noticed a light was still coming from Nancy's room. He glanced at the digital clock on his night stand and noted that it was 2:00 A.M. She must have fallen asleep reading, he reasoned, and decided to quietly go in and shut it off so as not to disturb her. He fumbled for his light switch, slithered out of bed and headed for Nancy's room without bothering to put on his slippers. At first glance he thought she was still awake as her eyes were open. But then fear struck as he realized that both eyes were gazing off in the same direction and she lay absolutely motionless. Dear God, she's had a stroke he said to himself and his first and natural reaction was to cradle her in his arms trying to comfort her as tears streamed down his cheeks. "It's all right, darlin, it's all right" he kept repeating as the two of them rocked back and forth. Collecting himself somewhat he realized that this was not doing her a bit of good and that he had to get some professional help right away. He called 911.

Within fifteen minutes the paramedics arrived. Three of them, one female and two males, entered through the garage entrance carrying cases of medical supplies and pushing a collapsible gurney. And while by law they were not allowed to give any diagnoses they did agree with Bob that it certainly looked as if she had suffered a stroke. After a quick examination for traces of bleeding, broken bones or other serious trauma they lifted her upon the gurney and transported her to the Highland Park Hospital. Bob followed the ambulance to the hospital and stayed by Nancy's side constantly including during the admission process that eventually landed her in 1327 West a semi private room. The attending physician told Bob that she was resting comfortably and that there was nothing more they could do for her until the next morning. He suggested Bob go home and try to get some sleep. Still in a daze Bob did drive home, tidied up after the paramedics, made both his and Nancy's beds and went into the den and sat in the dark. This whole night had been incredulous. Prayer like thoughts kept running through his mind. Please, God, don't let her die. Don't take her away from me and the girls. Not just yet. What if she should die, what will I do? I can't live without her.

What if she has another stroke. I've heard they often come in pairs. My God, if that happened she'd be even worse than she is now. How could she possibly be worse than she is now…motionless and can't talk? Why did this have to happen to her… why not me instead? After tossing and turning in his La-Z Boy for what seemed to be for hours, he finally dropped off to sleep from sheer exhaustion.

When he awoke after a restless and very short sleep the sun was streaming through an east window and he thought about calling his daughters but then noticed by his watch that it was only 5:30 in the morning. He decided that if he called them now and got them out of bed at this hour the news would be twice as frightening for them. He decided to make a pot of coffee, fix some toast and call them later. The time seemed to drag but at 7:45 he decided to call them regardless. He dialed Meghan. Meghan is their first born and lives in Omaha with her husband Dave and their three year old son, Douglass Robert Campbell. Dave is in the real estate field and has done quite well for himself and his family. In four short years he has been 'salesman of the year' twice and promoted to assistant manager of commercial properties. Bob was reminded of the day Dave called to tell him and Nancy that they were now proud grandparents of a baby boy. The cycle of life he thought. God giveth and God taketh away. And now Nancy could be facing death. These macabre thoughts were interrupted when Meghan answered the phone.

"I hope I didn't wake you up", Bob said.

"What with a three year old," she chuckled. "How are you, Dad?" She and her dad quickly exchanged pleasantries and Bob wasted no time in passing along the sad news about her mother.

"I'm coming to Deerfield right away, Dad. I'll call you after I make flight arrangements. Will you be able to meet me at the airport, I hope?"

"No sweetheart. It won't be necessary. There's nothing you can do to help at this point. I'll call you everyday to give you progress reports. It's going to be a very long road back and there will be plenty of time for you to visit her once she comes home. In the meantime pray for her speedy recovery." After some bickering Meghan reluctantly agreed and asked if he would like her to call Elizabeth for him. He thanked her but said it was something he had to do.

The phone call to Elizabeth was nearly a carbon copy of that to Meghan. Elizabeth lives with her husband Frazier in Elgin, Illinois. They have been married for only a couple of years and rent a two bedroom apartment. Since graduating from Northern Illinois University, where they met, they have both been concentrating on improving their financial position to a point where thoughts of raising a family might become a reality. Frazier earned a master in business administration and for now is working for a small manufacturing firm that makes small parts for the automotive industry. After a short conversation and after both had hung up the phone Bob gave a big sigh of relief. That difficult ordeal was thankfully over.

For the next few days Nancy underwent a prescribed regimen of physical therapy to reeducate the muscles needed for walking and talking. Bob was at her side constantly and even assisted in helping with the physical therapy exercises. He stayed with her every waking moment and even had his meals in the hospital cafeteria. The recovery progress was agonizingly slow and it simply ripped him apart to see her pitifully incontinent and lose control of all body functions. After four days of almost perpetual care Nancy suffered another stroke, lapsed into a coma and passed away a day and a half later. Bob was so upset that the hospital staff had someone drive him safely home. His worst fear had become a reality. His beloved Nancy was gone.

Chapter 2

THE MEMORIAL

Bob knew what he had to do although he didn't want to. It will be one of the most difficult things he has ever done. But the girls must be told now. To avoid going through the torture twice, he arranged a conference call between the three of them. When all three were connected on line Bob opened the discussion with a weak and trembling voice.

"Girls, I have some very bad news. Your mother suffered another stroke which proved to be too much for her to handle and she has died." His voice was barely audible at the end and when Meghan and Elizabeth started to cry he was no longer able to control his emotions and began to weep out loud himself. Eventually each one gained enough control to carry on a somewhat intelligible conversation.

"Have you made any arrangements yet, Dad?" asked Meg.

"And what can we do to help?" Liz followed up.

"Nothing really except coming home for the memorial if you can get away. A few years ago your mom and I made final arrangements with the Neptune Society to be cremated. They handle everything…all the details. They pick up the body, wherever it might be – even out of the country – cremate it and dispose of the ashes in accordance with family wishes. Your mother said she wanted my ashes delivered to her and I made a promise to keep hers as well should she precede me in death. So you see everything is well under control from that standpoint. All that is left for me to do is make arrangements for a memorial service and the Reverend Thorp has assured me that he will relieve me of that responsibility totally. And that's a big load off my mind."

"How are you holding up, Dad?" Liz asked.

"Oh, I'm doing okay, I guess. I've got some solace in the fact that she is no longer incapacitated or incontinent and doesn't have to face a long uphill battle back to some semblance of normalcy. But then it's the finality of it all that is so difficult to handle."

"When is the memorial service?" Meg asked.

"It's set for Wednesday two weeks from tomorrow. That should give you both enough time to put things in order before you come. If Dave and Frazier can get away that would be fine – we have plenty of room here. And I'm certain we could find someone to stay with Douglass during the service if you think it would be inappropriate or too mystifying for him to be in the church. I shall wait to hear from you both once you've made your arrangements." They all said their 'goodbyes' and ended a most stressful conference call.

There was a small mournful gathering at the Deerfield Community Church seated behind Bob Holt, his two daughters and their husbands for a memorial service honoring the life of Nancy Holt. Several people rose to pay homage to her and remark about what a loving wife and mother she was. Some mentioned that outside the home she was very active in civic and church activities. One lady rose to deliver an anecdote about Nancy trying to get out of a sand trap at a golf course. It seems she took three or four swipes at the ball which each time hit the lip of the trap and rolled back in. Finally in frustration she picked the ball up and threw it onto the green. That story seemed to loosen up the crowd a bit and others were more willing to stand up and talk about Nancy. All in all nine people stood to pay tribute to her. After a moving service by Reverend Thorp, a reception was held in the fellowship hall of the church where a small lunch and refreshments were served.

It was well after 1:00 P.M. when Bob and his family final got home – mentally fatigued more than physically tired. It had been an exhausting day but one that Nancy would have appreciated very much. Dave and Frazier had to leave early to get back to their jobs but the girls stayed on to be with their dad and lend support for a couple of days. Frazier dropped Dave at the airport and then drove home to Elgin. Bob and his daughters were relaxing in the den reflecting on all the events of the past few days. Meg and Liz had usurped both of the La-Z Boy chairs, dropped their shoes on the floor and leaned back in comfort. Bob stretched out on a couch with a double bourbon highball. The ladies were sipping some sherry wine. Finally he broke the silence and said:

"Girls before you leave for home I would like your help in the disposition of your mother's things. She and I talked a little about this from time to time and I have an idea what some of her wishes were but other than that I'm lost and need input from both of you."

"But Dad,Liz interjected, isn't a little early to be thinking about that? Mom's been gone only a few days. There's plenty of time for that later when we will all be better prepared mentally to handle it. I really don't think I could bear it just now."

"Believe me, Liz, I don't relish the idea anymore than you but I guess it's best in the long run to remove all things so that you aren't constantly reminded of your loss. I can understand that. I know it would bother me to see your Mom's things lying around always reminding me that she's gone for good and that I'll never be able to see or touch her again."

"I've heard the same thing, Meg added, after all Dad you'll always have your pleasant memories of her – they can never take those away."

"Amen to that, Meg."

"Okay with me, I guess. How can we be of help?" Liz asked.

"Well, I know that she had promised her wedding ring to you, Meg. She also mentioned that she would like you, Liz, to have her diamond engagement ring as well as the Sterling silver tea set. And I believe there's enough Sterling silverware for each of you to have place settings for six. As for her Rolex watch, you can draw straws – or however you wish to decide. Beyond that I don't know of any specific requests she had for the two of you so I've laid out her things on one of the beds in the master bedroom and you can each take turns selecting what you'd like to have.

The girls spent the rest of the afternoon selecting mementos of their mother in full harmony without any disagreements or hard feelings. Bob rewarded them by taking them out to dinner at the 'Ye Ole Steak House' one of the nicest restaurants in town. Being with his daughters gave him pleasure, as it always did, but this time having them near was special consolation for his loss of Nancy. He was truly grateful for their support At one point during dinner he announced that on the following day they had a couple of closets to go through. He told them that what they didn't want would be given to the Salvation Army and Goodwill so they shouldn't be bashful or hesitant about choosing.

Much later after the girls had retired for the night and he was alone with his thoughts he walked down the hallway to the master bedroom and stood in the doorway staring at Nancy's bed. All of the events of the past few days ran through his mind like a rerun of a horror movie. Now, for the first time, the events began to anger him. He thought of the chiropractor she had gone to and wondered if his treatments could have caused her stroke – or maybe both of them. He recalled that their family physician, Dr. Stormont, had admonished them several times that chiropractic adjustments of the neck could cause a stroke. Yes, that's got to be it, he thought. I think I'll sue the bastard. With that final thought he turned away slowly and with misty eyes walked back down the hallway to the guestroom and went to bed. Sleep came surprisingly soon.

Chapter 3

TOM CLAYTON

Tom Clayton had become a well known and respected chiropractic physician in Deerfield, Illinois. He had always wanted to be a doctor. Even as a youngster he used to fantasize speeding through traffic to make house calls and saving lives. The privilege, if indeed it ever was one, of speeding through traffic making house calls has long since been abandoned by most physicians when it was discovered they could see more patients, and therefore make more income, by having patients come to them. The infamous waiting room was thus born and continues to this day as a bane to society exposing others to infectious diseases and imposing hardships upon many in getting to and from their offices. Waiting twenty, thirty sometimes forty five minutes or more for a doctor to spend maybe five minutes with you can be most aggravating to say the least. More responsible scheduling is often needed but deliberately ignored. It's all about money. Tom chose the chiropractic profession because like homeopaths and naturopaths he has a strong belief in the sanctity of Mother Nature and her resolute ability to help our bodies heal themselves. Tom was sitting at his desk on his day off going through his mail. He was separating journals and medical literature into one pile, bills into another and junk mail into file thirteen when he came across an envelope with a return address of Shane, Bailey and White, Inc., Attorneys at Law. Curiosity prompted him to open it immediately. He didn't like what he read at all:

"Dear Dr. Clayton:

Please be advised that we represent Mr. Robert Holt who claims you caused his wife, Nancy Holt, to incur a stroke and eventual death as a direct result of your chiropractic adjustments to her cervical spine. Mr. Holt is asking restitution in the amount of three million dollars ($3,000,000) in damages, pain and suffering.

Please contact us at your earliest opportunity regarding this matter.

Sincerely,
James White"

Stunned beyond belief Tom read and reread the letter each time with more disbelief and increasing anger. The world, he decided, was full of too many lazy people trying to get something for nothing. This is crazy, he thought. He knew that chiropractors all over the world performed literally thousands upon thousands of cervical adjustments every day without incident. The procedure has been around since 1898 when chiropractic was born and is widely used because it is perfectly safe. Malpractice has never been much of a threat to chiropractor during all those years and certainly shouldn't be now. Greed. That's what it is. Why can't people understand that these frivolous law suits demanding millions of dollars in settlements are a major cause of the higher cost of healthcare that we all face. Every year I have to increase the limit of my liability insurance and the premiums have increased dramatically. All these thoughts ran through his mind over and over again as he now paced back and forth in front of his desk.

When his tremors calmed down along with his heart palpations and he felt as if he was breathing somewhat normally, he reached for the phone and called his friend and lawyer Art Cummings. The firm of Foxford and Cummings has handled all his legal affairs for the practice as well as his personal matters since Tom opened his practice over twenty years ago. The receptionist put him straight through to Art.

"Good morning, Tom, how may I help you

"My God, Art, I'm being sued!"

"What for? Give me some of the details." Tom read him the letter from Shane,Bailey and White and waited for his reaction.

"Well, Tom I must say they are some of the most aggressive prosecutors in the State. I would imagine their success rate is well up into the nineties."

"Oh that's just dandy. Any other encouraging remarks you have for me?"

"Now Tom don't get upset. I wasn't trying to frighten you but simply let you know we will be facing a very formidable opponent. I'll give them a call right after we hang up identifying us as your representative and confirming it in writing. We should get together as soon as possible to discuss all the details and begin developing our defense. When can you free up an hour or so for a meeting?" After comparing calendars they agreed upon a date and time to meet at Art's office.

Tom decided to go home. The hell with the rest of the mail, he thought. The rest of it sure as hell couldn't be any worse than what he had gotten so far. He was mentally drained anyway as you might expect receiving a letter like that. He drove home half dazed and nearly missed stopping at two intersections. Fortunately for him they both were four way stops and no officers or surveillance cameras were lurking for violators. He thought some of stopping at a tavern for a drink but then thought better of it when he pictured himself in a bar before noon and being recognized by one of his patients. When he arrived home he spotted a note on the kitchen table from his wife June. It read that she was out shopping for groceries and would be home in time to make his lunch. He thought about having a drink to settle his nerves but noted by the kitchen wall clock that it still wasn't even noon yet. To hell with the time, I really need a drink to quiet my nerves, he rationalized. And so he poured himself a large glass of chardonnay and took it into the family room. He had just barely gotten comfortable in his favorite chair when June arrived home. He unloaded the rest of the groceries from the car and the two of them put them away into cupboards.

"Why are you drinking alcohol at this hour?" she asked.

"Maybe you'd better sit down. I have some bad news." They both pulled chairs out from under the kitchen table and sat across from one another. June had a perplexed and concern look about her. "I got a letter this morning from some attorneys informing me that I'm being sued by one of my patients' husband. He's claiming that I caused his wife to have a stroke as a result of a cervical adjustment and he wants three million dollars in damages. I guess he means to bring a malpractice suit against me. Isn't that ducky, though?"

"No, it's just awful, that what it is." What are you going to do?"

" I've already called my lawyer. You remember Art Cummings, June. He and his wife were at our open house last Christmas." June nodded. "I've got an appointment with him next week to sort things out and plan a defense. It's going to be settled in court for sure." Tom poured himself another glass of wine. June moved close and gave him a big reassuring hug and said that she knew he would weather this storm just like he had all the others in the past.

"It seems incredulous that anyone would do such a thing. It doesn't seem fair after you've spent twenty some odd years caring for people, even making house calls on a Sunday, to have someone turn against you like this. It's terrible how a few dollars can so completely change a person.

"I don't call three million a few dollars", Tom said. "If I didn't have any insurance, I'd be wiped out."

"It was just a figure of speech, honey. What does Art have to say?"

"As I mentioned I'm going to see him early next week to plan our strategy. He says the law firm of Shane, Bailey and White is one of the sharpest in the State and that their prosecution success rate is very high – in the nineties he said. He indicated that we must prove to a jury that my treatments couldn't have possibly caused Nancy to have a stroke. After all I treated her last month and here it is April before she had a stroke. That time delay, I would think, would certainly play in my favor. I'm confident that we'll win this thing but until we do it's going to be a pain in the you know what. The more I think about it the angrier I become with Mr.Holt" Tom poured yet another glass of chardonnay.

"That's not going to solve anything," June said looking toward the wine bottle.

"I know it but it sure as hell helps me deal with it right now. Maybe before I get too thick tongued and incoherent I'd better give the kids a call and let them know their father is accused of murder."

"Now Tom don't make light of this. It's serious business. You could be found guilty, ya know." Tom reached for the wall phone on the kitchen wall and dialed the number for Jenny who is in her last year at Illinois University and studying for a masters degree in business administration.

"Hello she answered.

"Hi darlin, this is your dad. How are you?" Before she could answer he continued, "Not studying any human anatomy with some of the boys from the fraternities, I hope."

"TOM!!" scolded June.

"No Dad. I remember those admonishing lectures of yours only too well. Are you checking up on me or is there another reason you're calling in the middle of the day?"

"We do have a small bit of disturbing news. The husband of a former patient of mine is suing me for malpractice, It seems his wife suffered two strokes and died and he is claiming it was due to my adjustments. I just wanted you to know about it and that your mother and I are not at all concerned about the eventual outcome although it's certainly going to be a pain in the ass until it's over. Here say a hello to your mom." He handed the phone to June and headed for the family room with another glass of wine and simply relax knowing that no two women could just chat on the phone for a few minutes. And he was right. June didn't join him for another thirty minutes.

"Did you girls get all talked out?"

"Yes we did and Jenny wanted me to tell you that she feels very badly about your predicament and hopes it becomes resolved real soon."

"That was nice of her. I appreciate it." Tom then used the phone on the desk in the family room to call their son, Bill who was also away at school. He had received his bachelor of science degree in human biology from the University of Illinois and is now in his second year at National College of Chiropractic in Lombard, Illinois. Although he would never pressure him, Tom hopes that after graduation Bill would come in with him and eventually take over his practice when he retired.

"Hi son, what are you doing in the dorm at 2:30 in the afternoon – not cutting class I hope?"

"No, but I've got a neuroanatomy class at 3:00 that I'd LIKE to cut though. How are you and Mom?"

"Oh we're fine. Neuroanatomy, heh. Yeah it was a tough course for me too. I'll never forget the first quiz we had on the central nervous system. Your dad got a big fat zero! I didn't know the lentiform nucleus from the hypothalamus."

"I'll be sure to watch out for that one, Dad. What's up?" Tom repeated the same information he had given to Jenny and once again turned the phone over to June who's conversation this time would be constrained due to Bill's 3:00 o'clock class schedule. After Bill's phone call June ambled over to the wet bar in the corner of the family room, mixed a martini straight up with an onion and joined Tom on the couch.

"Well, Tom said, this has certainly been a day and a half, hasn't it? No patients, being sued, incurred the promise of legal fees that I can't afford and probably will have another increase in insurance premiums. Keeps one on his toes, doesn't it?"

"Yup, it sho do." June replied as they touched glasses.

Chapter 4

THE PRETRIAL MEETING

Art Cummings entered the reception room directly from his office and greeted Tom Clayton. After exchanging pleasantries Art led him down a long hallway lined with private offices to their posh conference room.. In the center of the room stood a very large solid oak table that easily seated twelve persons comfortably and possibly as many as sixteen in a pinch. All chairs, including those placed around the perimeter, were cushioned and armed. There is only one entryway consisting of two ten foot high solid wooden doors situated centrally along one wall. There are no windows in the room that might distract from any business proceedings and on the wall directly opposite the entryway is a large portrait of the founder of the firm, Bertram James Foxford, affectionately known by his close friends and colleagues as 'B.J.'. Also hanging on all walls were assorted paintings interspersed with photographs and awards all decoratively arranged. A wall to wall beige berber carpeting finished off a comfortable and pleasant place to conduct business. Art sat at one end of the huge table with Tom seated to his right and a stenographer, Ms. Gordon, to the left. Between them was a silver tray containing a pot of coffee, some china cups and a small plate of assorted pastries. A pad of paper and pen were supplied for Tom's use but Art typically used a legal sized yellow pad.

Art opened the meeting by asking Tom if there were any new developments since they last talked.

"None that I can think of at the moment," Tom said. "I assume you have informed Shane, Bailey and White that you are representing me."

"We have, yes. And we received an acknowledgement letter from them. James White will be prosecuting the case for them. How long had Mrs. Holt been a patient of yours?"

"About two years."

"How often did she visit your office?"

"About once a month. She said she liked to come in for her 'tune ups'. Once in a while she would cancel an appointment but all in all she was a very steady patient.

"When was the last time you saw her – professionally that is?"

"March 25th."

"Did you adjust her cervical vertebrae at that time?"

"Yes."

"So you have adjusted them for a total 25 times or there abouts. Is that correct?"

"At least that many, yes."

"To your knowledge, Tom, had she ever experienced any kind of an adverse reaction to one of your treatments?"

"No."

"Have ANY of your patients suffered any type of adverse reaction to treatments – a headache, nausea, anything like that?"

"None that I am aware of."

"Have you always employed the same techniques and procedures on your patients?"

"Yes on all my patients. I've always used the techniques that I learned at the National College of Chiropractic which is a fully accredited institution."

"Can an adjustment to the neck be dangerous?"

"No more than adjustments to other areas of the spine. That's especially true if they are performed by a licensed practitioner and not by a physical therapist or masseuse. If it were dangerous, we wouldn't do it."

"What could make it a dangerous practice?"

"One must be careful not to put the head into extension while abruptly rotating it to one side or the other. That raises the possibility, remote as it is, that the vertebral artery could be compromised in such a way as to decrease the flow of blood to the brain."

"Has this ever happened?"

"I've never heard of it myself nor have I ever read any report to that effect. This idea of creating a stroke by adjusting the cervical vertebrae is a myth perpetrated and perpetuated by the medical profession in an effort to discredit our profession. Medical doctors really don't like others in the health care profession that are not under their direct control. And that's especially true if they represent an economic treat to them as we do. They don't like us being the second largest health care profession and for years have called us quacks, and an unscientific cult among other demeaning slanders."

"Didn't I read something about a law suit that chiropractors won against them?" Art asked.

"You did. It was a discrimination suit against the AMA," Art said he would review that case to see if we could use any of it to our advantage. Then he asked Tom to explain how the prosecution could make a case out of cervical adjustments causing a stroke.

"Cervical vertebrae are unique in that an artery, the vertebral artery, travels closer to the bones in the neck than anywhere else along the spine. Six of the seven bones in the neck have a small opening on each side called a foramen. The vertebral arteries – one on each side – pass through these foramina on their way to the brain. Medical doctors contend that moving a neck bone narrows these openings and compromises blood flow to the brain."

"In your opinion, Tom, what would the odds be of this ever happening?"

"They would be astronomical. There are about 60,000 chiropractors in the country. If each of them adjusted only ten necks a day for a five day week and forty week year – well you do the math. It would be around a hundred and twenty million adjustments a year.

"Do you know of other chiropractors using the same cervical techniques as you?"

"Art, an adjustment is a very slight movement of a bone that is misaligned with another. This is called a subluxation. One doctor might move the bone with a thumb contact while another would choose to use a finger contact. But their objective is the same. So techniques are basically the same but the contacts can vary."

"I think those are all the questions I have for you today, Tom. But I want you to know that a malpractice suit is very very difficult to prove. It must be shown that a practitioner willfully uses or used and instrument or procedure not recognized, accepted and in general use by other comparable practitioners. Unfortunately lawyers have drifted away from the malpractice concept and have developed convincing arguments for juries that just mistakes by physicians are worth millions of dollars to their clients. And they, the lawyers, charge a third of any settlement. It's real big business! So, what I'm saying is that we have to concentrate our defense upon the premise that your cervical adjustments could not have possibly caused Mrs. Holt's stroke.

The session with Art lasted longer than Tom had anticipated and when he returned to the office the waiting room was loaded with patients. He immediately put the law suit out of his mind and spent the remainder of the day concentrating on sick people.

Chapter 5

THE TRIAL

In the days and weeks before the trial date both counselors were busy preparing their respective cases by lining up witnesses and coaching them while trying to anticipate potential exigencies and contingencies. On the first day of the trial nervous tensions abounded and were especially strong in Tom Clayton. He had never even seen the inside of a courtroom let alone becoming a defendant in one and everything about it gave him a very uneasy feeling and sense of anxiety. Being innocent until proven guilty didn't seem to help either. As the jury selection process progressed, though, he became a little more relaxed and increasingly more attentive and interested in the proceedings. One potential juror had been a patient of Dr. Clayton and of course challenged by the prosecution and was dismissed. Two others had had uncomfortable experiences with chiropractors outside of Illinois but were successfully challenged by Art Cummings anyway and were dismissed by the judge. All others were accepted without challenge. The completed jury was comprised of seven females, all housewives, and five males, two retired and three middle aged but still active in the workplace, after some prospective members had been challenged and dismissed because either the prosecution or defense counsel judged them to be biased to their case. Art said nothing to Tom for fear of compounding his tension but he was less than happy with a preponderance of females selected for the jury. He knew females by in large tend to be more emotional than males who tend to be more practically inclined. After the jury had been selected and the judge had retired to his chambers, family members from both sides were admitted into the courtroom for preferred seating near the front. June sat in the first row directly behind her husband who was seated at the table for the defense. Finally the Press and general visitors were admitted.

When all seating had been finished the bailiff called the court into session and announced that the Honorable Judge Justin O'Malley would be presiding. As if on cue he entered from a door to the left of the bench and made his way up to the elevated chair reserved for judges. He is a strikingly handsome man in his fifties, clean shaven and with just a suggestion of graying at the temples adding to his good looks. An imposing black robe enhanced his overall presence. He has a reputation of being somewhat strict but uncommonly fair. He swings a fair gavel, they say. These traits help keep him in popular demand by lawyers to hear their cases.

"Good morning everyone," he said and then looked toward the prosecutions table. "Mr. White does the prosecution wish to make an opening statement?"

"We do your honor," James White responded as he rose from his chair and approached the jury box. "Ladies and gentlemen of the jury we will prove conclusively that Mrs. Holt died of a stroke as a direct result of a chiropractic adjustment to her neck administered by the defendant." He turned toward Tom Clayton and pointed at him with a stiff arm. "We will show how a chiropractic adjustment of the neck by forcefully moving a bone can shut down the blood supply to the brain leading to a stroke. You will have experts explain in simple terms how this happened to Mrs. Holt. I ask you why do chiropractors adjust bones at all? I submit that it is totally unnecessary. They talk of misalignments of the spine. You all look fine sitting there. Is your spine misaligned? I don't think so. I stand up and walk straight without limping. Is my spine misaligned? No it isn't. Mr. Clayton is no doctor. He's merely an incompetent bone crusher." Again James White turned a pointed a straight arm at Tom turned only his head back toward the jury and said, "This man has taken a loved one away from a husband and two lovely daughters as a result of his poor practice of chiropractic and total lack of understanding the consequences of his actions. His incompetence has left a huge void in the Holt family. He should be on trial for murder and not simply malpractice. My client is asking you to award a settlement of three million dollars in damages pain and suffering." James White returned to his seat at the prosecution table.

"Mr. Cummings, does the defense have an opening statement?"

"We do your honor." Art Cummings made his way to the jury box and with a smile on his face nodded a couple of times toward the jury. "Ladies and gentlemen of the jury," he started, "it is blatantly obvious that the prosecution knows little or nothing about the honored profession of chiropractic and to overshadow their ignorance have resorted to character assassination. You should rebuke such an underhanded approach. We don't intend to dignify Mr. White's commentthat our client should be on trial for murder with any comment of our own. Instead we will present a short but factual course in chiropractic. Chiropractic physicians and their adjustments are concerned with things called subluxations. A complete dislocation of a joint is known as a luxation. However, a minor misalignment of two adjacent bones is called a subluxation – something far less than a dislocation. Most subluxations, in fact, can not be identified even on x-ray. In other words during a chiropractic adjustment the bones are moved only slightly – certainly not sufficiently enough to pinch an artery and interfere with the flow of blood. During his opening statement Mr. White accused my client of 'poor practice' implying malpractice. In order to be classified as malpractice it must be proven, not simply suggested, that Dr. Clayton willfully used an instrument or procedure that is not generally accepted or recognized and not in general use by other chiropractic physicians. My client's treatments of Mrs. Holt DO NOT fall into this classification. We will demonstrate beyond any doubt that Dr. Clayton, a physician with twenty years experience, could not have possibly caused Mrs. Holt to have a stroke. Thank you."

"It's been a long and trying day," the judge interjected," selecting a jury and hearing open arguments. We will resume tomorrow morning at 9:00 o'clock. Court is adjourned." A rap of the gavel sent nearly everyone scurrying for the exit. All except Art Cummings who asked Tom to stay over for a few minutes because he had some questions. They were still seated at the defense table and as Art put papers back into his brief case he turned to Tom and asked about the prosecutions emphasis on pinching an artery as the cause of a stroke.

"We talked about this during our pretrial meeting and I got the impression that it was a rarity – no big deal. It sounds as if White intends it to be the center of his case against us," he said.

"Art, he was alluding to the vertebral arteries. Remember I mentioned that there is one on each side of the cervical spine. They come off the subclavian artery and course through a transverse foramen , a small opening within a portion of the bone. They travel through foramina in six of the seven cervical vertebrae and finally enter a large foramen at the base of the skull and hence to the brain. White's contention that rotating the head and moving a bone in the neck at the same time can effectively make a foramen small enough to compromise the artery passing through it."

"Has this ever been demonstrated as with cineography for example?"

"Not to my knowledge. As you pointed out in your opening remarks most subluxations can't even be seen on an x-ray let alone see them moving."

"I see. Then it is important to THEIR case and not ours. I would rather imagine that White will introduce it again – possibly with an expert witness of some sort. We'd better be ready for it, anyway."

June heard Tom pull into the garage and met him at the side door. They kissed and hugged longer than usual.

"Mmm you feel good to me, honey."

"You do as well. Tough day in court?"

"Not really. A lot of the time was spent selecting a jury. That was before you arrived. But this whole damned thing has gotten me up tight and that's exhausting, ya know?"

"Were you nervous? "

"At first, yes. Very. But then after a bit I settled down. Didn't enjoy it, mind you, just a little more at ease. How was your day before you came to the court?"

"Routine. Did a little dusting and vacuuming. Oh, and I made your favorite cookies."

"Good, maybe I can bribe the jury with them." Hear anything from either one of our urchins today?"

"Nothing yet today. I've got an idea Tom. Why don't you whip up a pitcher of martinis, we'll go out on the porch and you can tell me how lovely I am and how much you love me."

"Great idea. Why didn't I think of that?"

Shortly before 9:00 the next morning Art and Tom were settling in at their table in the courtroom and Art kept glancing at Tom.

"Are you all right, Tom? You look like hell. What did you do spend the night in a bar?"

"No nothing like that. June and I split a pitcher of martinis is all."

31

"Followed by a little lovin, maybe?"

"That falls under doctor/patient confidentiality, Art."

"Uh huh," Art said with broad smirk on his face.

"All rise," bellowed the bailiff. "The Honorable Judge Justin O'Malley presiding." At that point June entered the courtroom and took a seat behind the defense counsel's table.

"Good morning everyone", the judge said. "Mr. White call your first witness."

"The prosecution calls Mr. Holt." Bob Holt nonchalantly rose from his chair at the prosecution table and strolled to the witness chair. He was sworn in and asked to take a seat.

"Mr. Holt please describe for this court the series of events leading up to the untimely death of your wife."

"Well it was April 5th and Nancy and I were getting ready to retire. She said she was pretty tired and thought she would start locking up and shutting off lights. I decided to watch the rest of the 10:00 o'clock news. When I finally got into bed and shut off the light I noticed a light coming from her room. I figured she was reading in bed, a favorite pastime of hers. I woke up about 2:00 in the morning – at this point Bob began to have difficulty forming words and his eyes became misty – and note… noticed her light was still on. I wen… went to her room and there she was-just lying motionless." Now tears began running down his cheeks. He lowered his head and dried the tears as best he could with his hand trying to hide his embarrassment. Then James White interrupted:

"Take your time, Mr. Holt. There's no hurry. I know this must be very difficult for you but your testimony is important. Please continue only when you feel up to it." There was a few minute pause while Bob Holt reached for a couple of facial tissues from a box on the corner of the bench, dried his tears once again, quietly blew his nose and composed himself sufficiently to continue.

"I'm sorry," he said softly. "That's about all I can tell you. She laid motionless staring off to the right with both eyes. I finally called 911 and the paramedics took her to the Highland Park Hospital."

"When did you realize your wife had had a stroke?" Art Cummings stood up immediately and cried:

"Objection! It calls for a conclusion on the part of the witness."

"Overruled, I'll allow it. The witness may answer."

"I only guessed that it was a stroke when I saw her lying there not moving and staring at the wall. The paramedics refused to tell me anything officially and it was the intern at the hospital that confirmed my suspicions."

"Had your wife ever experienced anything like that before? Maybe like a transient ischemic attack or light headedness?"

"No."

"Did she fall or have some type of blow to her head"

"No."

"But she was in the habit of receiving chiropractic treatments wasn't she?"

"Yes, she went to a chiropractor just about every month. Dr. Clayton there," he looked toward and pointed at Tom Clayton as he spoke.

"Did she ever have any kind or adverse reaction to any of Dr. Clayton's treatments?"

"She never complained but I thought several times that she acted a little light headed."

"In what way?"

"Well she seemed to be a little unsteady on her feet at times."

"I see. You mean like when you get up very suddenly you get kind of dizzy from the lack of blood to the brain?"

"Objection!"

"Withdrawn. I have no further questions, your honor." Jim White walked back to his seat and the judge asked if the defense wished to cross examine.

"We do your honor. Mr. Holt please except our deepest sympathy over the loss of your wife. We realize how agonizing this must be for you and I promise to be as brief as possible."

"Thank you," he whispered.

"Was your wife taking any medication, Mr. Holt?" James White sprang to his feet.

"Objection! Mrs. Holt is not on trial here."

"Your honor," Art replied, " the cause of Mrs. Holt's stroke is paramount to our defense."

"Overruled. The witness will answer the question." Art repeated the question for the witness.

"She was taking medication for a heart condition."

"What kind of heart condition?"

"She would sometimes experience an irregular heart beat."

"Do you know the name of the medication, Mr. Holt?"

"Yes, it's called Quinidine."

"Was she taking any other medication?"

"Yes, she was also on beta blockers for her blood pressure and occasionally she would take an antacid for heartburn. But nothing else."

"Thank you. That'll be all for now." The judge dismissed Bob Holt and instructed James White to call his next witness.

"We call Dr. John Richards to the stand." He was sworn in and took a seat in the witness chair.

" You are an intern at the Highland Park Hospital, is that correct?"

"No, actually I'm a resident there."

"I apologize, doctor, I was misinformed. What is your specialty?"

" Internal medicine."

"On the night of April 5th did you treat Mrs. Holt?"

"Yes."

" Were you able to diagnose her condition?"

"Yes she had suffered a stroke."

"Were you able to determine the cause?"

"No not specifically. A stroke results from a lack of blood to a portion of the brain. It is usually due to a blockage of a small blood vessel or a ruptured one."

"What treatment did you provide for Mrs. Holt?"

"There wasn't much we could do for her at that point. We put her on a blood thinner and gave her a sedative to help her sleep."

"Thank you doctor, I have no more questions. Your honor, we offer the hospital records for Mrs. Holt as exhibit A." The judge nodded and said they would be recorded.

"Cross, Mr. Cummings?"

"Yes your honor. Doctor would a fibrillating heart be considered as an irregular beat?"

"Yes it would."

"Could a fibrillating heart create enough turbulence to form a clot?"

"Definitely."

"And such a clot could travel to the brain and cause a blockage, could it not?"

"Yes, that would be one way to create a stroke."

"Thank you, nothing further."

"Redirect your honor?" asked James White.

"Doctor isn't there normal turbulence within the vascular system due to its frequent branching and tortuous paths?"

"Yes, but…

"That will be all doctor, thank you." We now call Dr. Byron Salter to the stand."

"You are a medical doctor, is that correct?"

"It is."

"Would you please describe your credentials to the jury."

"I graduated from Illinois University Medical School, served two years internship at Cook County Hospital, completed four years of residency in cardiology also at Cook County and have been in practice for fifteen years – specializing in cardiology."

"Is it correct to assume, then, that you have seen many cases of stroke patients?"

"Yes, more than I would care to."

"In your expert opinion could a chiropractic adjustment of a cervical vertebra cause a pinching of one of the vertebral arteries interfering with blood flow to the brain and cause a stroke?"

"If it was forceful enough, I guess it could."

"Your witness, Mr. Cummings." Art rose and stood by his chair and asked:

"Dr. Salter, have you ever seen this demonstrated such as on cineography?"

"No I have not."

"Then you have seen no proof that this could happen, is that correct?"

"Yes that would be correct." Art thanked him and sat down.

"Redirect your honor," James White requested.

"Proceed."

"Doctor, just because you haven't seen evidence of a chiropractic adjustment compromising a vertebral artery, doesn't mean it hasn't been witnessed by other experts does it?"

"Of course not."

"Thank you." In the absence of further questions from the defense, the judge dismissed the witness.

"Call you next witness, Mr. White."

"Your honor, the prosecution rests"

"Does the defense wish to call any witnesses?"

"We call Dr. Dan Stormont"

"May we approach your honor?" asked James White. The judge motioned both counselors to the bench and promptly shut off the microphone.

"The prosecution was not advised of this witness, White said. "we have not had time to prepare."

"It's getting rather late and it's a Friday. Would Monday morning give you enough time to prepare?"

"Yes that would be adequate, Judge, thank you." The judge turned the microphone back on and announced that the trial would resume on Monday morning at 9:00 o'clock.

After the court was called into session by the bailiff and the judge had been seated and called for order by rapping the gavel, he said "Good morning everyone. I trust you all had a pleasant weekend. We will begin today with witnesses for the defense. Mr. Cummings call your first witness please."

"We call Dr. Dan Stormont." A short, heavy set man approached, was sworn in and plumped down into the witness chair. "Doctor, you are the family physician for the Holt family, is that correct?"

"Yes."

"For how long?"

"I would say at least fifteen years."

"Mr. Holt testified that his wife had been taking Quinidine for an irregular heart beat. Did you prescribe that for her?"

"Yes I did."

"For how long a period had she been taking Quinidine?"

"Approximately five years."

"Then may we assume she was being helped by the medication?"

"Yes she was."

"Did you also prescribe beta blockers to lower her blood pressure?"

"Yes."

"And how long was she on those?"

"Also for about five years."

"Did you also prescribe antacids for her heartburn?"

"No. She must have gotten those over the counter at a pharmacy or maybe from another doctor."

"I see. Is it true that Quinidine can itself sometimes cause the heart to beat irregularly?"

"Yes it can. That's why it's so important to monitor the patients."

"Could that have been the case with Mrs. Holt?"

"Objection, your honor. It calls for a conclusion on the part of the witness,"James White said as he remained seated.

"Sustained. The jury will disregard the last question," the judge ruled.

"How often did you monitor Mrs. Holt's dosage of Quinidine?"

"I would say about every two to three months."

"That infrequently, doctor, even though she also taking Beta blockers and antacids?"

"Objection. Counsel is badgering the witness."

"Withdrawn," art said. "Thank you doctor, that will be all."

"Does the prosecution wish to cross examine?"

"No, your honor. We have no questions for this witness."

"Then call you next witness, Mr. Cummings," the judge directed.

"We call Dr. Tom Clayton." Tom turned around and gave June a quick kiss and he smiled at the jury as he passed them on the way to the witness chair.

"How long have you been a chiropractic physician, Dr. Clayton?"

"A little over twenty years."

"Please tell the court about the education required to become a chiropractor."

"Like most other medical schools it is a five year course – four years of classroom and laboratory study and one year internship."

"Internship? Do you intern in hospitals?"

"No in our own clinics associated with our colleges. We have been banned from hospitals by the AMA."

"Objection," James White called.

"Sustained. Just answer the questions, doctor," the judge ordered.

"Yes, sir. I apologize."

"The jury will disregard the last comment by the witness. Continue, Mr. Cummings."

"What courses are required for graduation?"

"We take the same course and use the same textbooks as medical students with the exception of pharmacology and surgery."

"Every state requires that chiropractors be licensed. What are those requirements?"

"There are boards that we must pass and in addition each state has it's own licensing examinations. After licensing most sates also require continual medical education to keep it in force."

"Mrs. Holt was a patient of yours?"

"Yes."

"For how long?"

"About two years?"

"During her visits to your office did you adjust her spine?"

"Yes during every visit."

"Did these adjustments include the cervical vertebrae?"

"Yes, they did."

"How many times would you say that you treated her over the two year period?"

"She came in about once a month so it would be twenty five or so treatments."

"When was the last time you treated her?"

"It was on March 25th."

"You heard testimony that Mrs. Holt didn't suffer a stroke until April 5th. Are you certain March 25th was the last time you treated her?"

"I am positive."

"Did Mrs. Holt ever have any kind of adverse reaction to one of your treatments?"

"None that I am aware of."

"You never noticed her being light headed, unstable or wobbly after one of your treatments?"

"No."

"Have you ever noticed any such reaction with ANY of your patients.?"

"Never from a spinal adjustment. I have had only two patients that began to show signs of going into shock while being treated with acupuncture."

"Do you have any knowledge, first hand or otherwise, of a chiropractor anywhere in the world having caused a stroke by adjusting cervical vertebrae?"

"I do not. The odds of it occurring are astronomical."

"Thank you, doctor. Nothing further."

"Does the prosecution have any questions for this witness,?" the judge asked.

"No, your honor."

"We will take a thirty minute recess before hearing the summations." The judge rapped the gavel, rose from his chair and retreated to his chambers.

Almost to the second Judge O'Malley returned to the courtroom thirty minutes later and called for the defense's summation. Art Cummings rose from his chair and was buttoning two of the three buttons of his suit coat as he approached the jury.

"Ladies and gentlemen this trial has been a waste of your valuable time and I do apologize for our part in it. Dr. Clayton didn't cause Nancy Holt to have a stroke. The prosecution has not produced one shred of evidence to prove that my client had anything to do with it. Dr. Clayton last treated Mrs. Holt on March 25th but she didn't suffer a stroke until April 5th. That's eleven days later! Eleven days in which she may very well had had a fibrillating heart that generated a clot that found its way to the brain. That's more feasible than a pinched artery eleven days earlier, don't you think? It is very unlikely that any decrease in blood supply to the brain would take eleven days to cause any kind of reaction such as a stroke. A deficient blood flow to the brain will always have an immediate affect. The expert witnesses that testified here today don't know the specific cause of Mrs. Holt's stroke either. They all spoke in generalities – nothing specific in Mrs. Holt's case. Chiropractors in this country perform over 100 million cervical adjustments every year and have for many years. Wouldn't you think that if it was a cause of stroke we would have heard or read about it by now? This is clearly not a case of malpractice and certainly not murder. No, this whole thing is a blatant attempt to filch money from an insurance company. Your money and mine. Your choice is clear. Because of a lack of sufficient evidence to prove any guilt the law demands that you must find my client not guilty. Thank you." Art returned to his place at the defense table and James White took his place addressing the jury.

"Ladies and gentlemen, I don't think this has been a waste of your time – or mine. How many strokes caused by chiropractic adjustments have gone unreported? Who knows? I certainly don't. But I do know that if there were more concerned people such as my client who is brave enough to come forward and call attention to this problem we might have a more accurate idea as to its magnitude. You have heard experts describe the vertebral arteries passing through tiny holes in cervical vertebrae in the neck. You've heard testimony that rotating the head and forcing one of the bones in the neck at the same time could compromise the flow of blood to the brain. No one has seen this on cineography that we know of, but no one has ever seen electromagnetic waves either. But we know what electromagnetic waves can do and now we know what rotating the head and forcing a cervical bone can do. You therefore should find Dr. Clayton guilty of malpractice. Thank you." James White went back to the table for the prosecution and sat down.

Judge O'Malley turned his chair so that he was directly facing the jury. ""Ladies and gentlemen you have heard the evidence. It becomes your duty now to determine the guilt or innocence of Dr. Clayton in the matter involving Mrs. Holt. The ball is in your court. No pun intended. You must weigh the evidence with as much impartiality and lack of bias as possible. You have a serious task in front of you. Don't hurry it. Vote your convictions based upon fact and not emotion. If you have any doubt you must find the defendant innocent. Thank you for your service. The bailiff will now lead you to a conference room for your deliberations."

The conference room was small but comfortable. Attendants were on hand to not only assure no one left the room without an escort but to serve them with food and drinks as well. Juror #5 was elected foreman as she had served on a jury previously. The next order of business was to take an initial vote. Voting, of course, was by secret ballot and all jurors were supplied with pencils and ample precut ballots. The voting results were tallied by the foreman by opening each one separately and announcing to the group guilty or not guilty. The result of the first ballot was four guilty and eight not guilty. The foreman then opened the discussions by stating that no evidence had been submitted that ANY chiropractor had ever caused a stroke. Juror #9 brought up the delay of eleven days between the last adjustment and the time Mrs. Holt suffered a stroke. Juror #4 alluded to the expert witnesses and their testimony that they thought it possible for a chiropractic adjustment of the spine in the neck to cause a stroke. And so it went for about an hour before the foreman asked for another vote. The result of this vote was two guilty and ten not guilty.

The jury was given a respite when a hot luncheon was served replete with rolls and butter and choice of beverage. There were only two or three engaged in conversations about the trial while the rest seemed satisfied to simply get acquainted with one another. When everyone had finished eating and the conference table had been cleared of dishes and remaining food the jurors assumed their original places at the table and deliberations were resumed. During the discussions that followed it became clear to everyone just who the two jurors were that continued to vote guilty. Art Cummings' concern was a valid one – both were females.

The word spread like wild fire. The jury is out after only two and a half hours of deliberations! When everyone was seated the jury filed into the courtroom followed closely by the judge.

"Has the jury reached a verdict?"

"We have your honor," replied the foreman. The foreman handed a folded sheet of paper with the verdict written on it to the bailiff who promptly delivered it to the judge. Judge O'Malley opened the sheet of paper, read the verdict and gave it back to the bailiff who then returned it to the foreman.

"Will the defendant please rise?" Both Tom Clayton and Art Cummings stood and remained at their places. "In the matter of Holt vs Clayton how do you find?" the judge asked.

"The jury finds the defendant, Dr. Thomas Clayton, not guilty," the foreman responded.

"Thank you ladies and gentlemen for your service," the judge said. "Dr. Clayton you are free to go. This court is adjourned." With a rap of the gavel members of the Press whipped out their cell phones and fled for the exit.

At home later June said she had made one of Tom's favorite dishes – chili and a toss salad with champagne pear vinaigrette with gorgonzola dressing. She asked if he wanted a cocktail before dinner or to just relax. He said that what he really wanted to do is take a long hot shower and wind down a bit. As he was rinsing the suds off when the shower door opened and June stepped in. She also showered herself and they thoughtfully washed one another's back. After toweling off Tom took June by the hand and led her into the bedroom and onto their bed.

"All rise," she giggled, the honorable Judge Clayton is unwinding!

Epilogue

In the weeks and months after the trial everyone's life seemed to take on a sense of normalcy, even for Bob Holt who was adjusting quite well to his loss of Nancy. In fact, he had even met a lovely woman that he was quite fond of and had seen on a few occasions. Jenny received her MBA and Bill was now an intern at National College of Chiropractic. Tom was kept busy at his practice which surprisingly had not diminished at all as a result of the trial publications. The number of new patients remained steady, if not at a slightly higher rate than usual. He told June he wasn't certain whether the new patients wanted his help or were simply curious to see him in person.

Today was like that. It was a Friday afternoon and as he made his way into one of his four treatment rooms he was astonished to see Bob Holt sitting at the end of an examining table.

"What can you do for congestive heart failure?" he asked.

PART TWO

First-hand anecdotes of chiropractic medicine are described. All names are fictional and any resemblance to actual names purely coincidental.

Chapter 6

Tom Clayton was certified in acupuncture several years ago and uses it in his practice on nearly every patient. He was drawn to it because of the very close correlation to chiropractic philosophy. Chiropractic doctrine holds that structure and function go hand in hand. If the body is structurally sound function will be normal and the body will heal itself. Acupuncturists, at least traditional ones, adhere to the tenet that if the energy within the basic energy pathways called meridians is balanced the body will heal itself. Both professions employ ancillary procedures such as vitamins, herbs, exercise, diet etc. This concept that the body's innate possesses the power to heal is a known fact often overlooked by orthodox medicine and completely disregarded by the pharmaceutical industry. Much to the publics misfortune. Although it is practiced in other countries and cultures, Tom was especially interested in the history behind Chinese acupuncture from whom we have learned the most about the art.

For many years in China acupuncture was practiced by families that developed secret formulas for all kinds of diseases and maladies and these formulas were passed on from generation to generation. This continued until Mao Tse Tung brought communism to China in the late forties. With communism everything is either controlled or run by a central government – food supply, transportation, communication, industrial output – everything. In keeping with this philosophy families practicing acupuncture were ordered to divulge their formulas. Although coercive and objectionable this did open up the art of acupuncture to the world. In doing so it was discovered that there was a striking similarity in the formulas. Most families had been treating the same diseases using identical acupuncture points. Although practiced in China for some five thousand years, acupuncture was not widely known and practiced in this country primarily due to bad press generated by orthodox medicine. Our erudite medical personnel consistently referred to it as an unscientific cult primarily because it didn't utilize patented drugs.

Bob Holt was still dangling his legs off the end of an examining table when he again said:

"Well, do you think you can do anything for my congestive heart condition?"

"I'm sure I can, Mr. Holt. I would like to try acupuncture. I've had some very good success with it in the past and if you're not in any great hurry I'd like to tell you about a most interesting and similar case to yours."

"I'm in no hurry. I'd like to hear it. How does acupuncture work anyway?" Tom pulled up a chair and began:

"The Chinese described 26 basic pathways of energy called meridians that run longitudinally around the body. There are twelve paired meridians, twelve and the right and twelve on the left sides of the body and two midline, one in front and one in back. These meridians are connected with one another and energy can be transferred from one to another. The meridians have never been seen either on gross or microscopic examination. But thanks to the radioactive studies performed by a Korean scientist, Kim Bong Han, their existence has been confirmed. Interestingly, it was found that the course of these meridians match up perfectly with those identified by the Chinese some 5000 years ago. Most of these energy pathways are directly associated with one of our internal organs and take their name from them. Accordingly, we have a lung meridian, a heart meridian, a large intestine meridian etc. The actual acupuncture points, the areas stimulated by a needle, electricity, temperature or pressure, are situated along the meridians' pathways. Not all meridians have the same number of stimulating points. Some have as few as eleven while the longest contains sixty- seven points. In cases of pain, especially of the musculoskeletal type, acupuncture stimulates or entices the body to produce and secrete powerful pain killing substances known as endorphins. Perhaps you have heard of them. They are hormones thought to be produced by the pituitary gland which is our master endocrine gland. At last count scientists have isolated some two hundred of them. There are quite a few of them as they appear to be rather specific in their actions. That is to say acupuncture points around a shoulder would be selected to signal the pituitary gland to produce and secrete endorphins specific for shoulder pain. I do know that one such endorphin was found to be fifty times more potent than morphine. Think of that! In the case of non-musculoskeletal diseases such as asthma, colitis, urinary infections, respiratory conditions and even heart conditions like yours, Mr. Holt, acupuncture works by balancing the energy within the meridians and letting the body heal itself."

"Is it painful?" Bob asked.

"That's a very common question and concern. The needles that I use are very thin. They are 35 gauge and look just like a small wire. Seriously, Mr. Holt, most of my patients never feel them. One time I was treating a patient with acupuncture who was lying on his stomach and after a few minutes he asked me what I was doing. He felt nothing at all. When I told him I was doing acupuncture he damned near died. Once in awhile a point might be a little sensitive and some experience a slight aching feeling – but no acute pain ever. Here I'll demonstrate." With that Tom inserted a one half inch, 35 gauge needle into his own forearm approximately two inches above the wrist – a point known as triple heater 5.

"Let me try it," Bob asked. Tom repeated the process. "Gee, you're right, I didn't feel a thing! Okay, when do we start?"

"See Barbara at the front desk on your way out. She'll set up an appointment for you. Mr. Holt you should be prepared to give this some quality time. Your heart condition didn't develop over night and it's not going to heal over night. If you are not willing to give it some time, I would recommend that you don't start. I can't give you a time frame. It might take as long as six months before we would see some results. Your breathing might become a little easier, maybe you'd have more energy and not tire so easily. Any sign would be encouragement enough to continue treatments At least at the start I would want to see you twice a week – anything less could be a waste of your time and money."

"I'm willing to give it time because my medical doctor hasn't done anything except tell me that the condition is progressive. Do you have some time now to tell me about the similar case you mentioned earlier?"

"Why don't you see Barbara first because she's probably getting ready to go home. I'll be in my office down the hall behind the reception desk." Bob Holt did as Dr. Clayton suggested and soon appeared at his office door. Tom waved him into the room and gestured to a lounge chair to the right of his desk. He then began:

"Jim G… first came to us with a neck problem. I have forgotten the nature of it but it was only necessary for him to be treated with chiropractic adjustments once or twice. We also treated him with acupuncture using many points on his back and along the spinal column. These points are known as the association points in that each one has a direct association with an internal organ. And stimulating these association points, then, moves energy through the meridians creating balance and allowing the body to utilize energy where it is needed to heal itself. After a couple of treatments Jim expressed a desire to come in once a month for one of these treatments. You see, they are very relaxing and euphoric to most patients. I can't recall the exact time period but after several months and at the conclusion of one of his sessions Jim asked if I would listen to his heart. I asked him what was wrong with his heart as he didn't mention anything during the taking of his history or physical examination. He stated that he had these "skips" during heart beats. Skips are often mistaken by patients for premature ventricular contractions or PVC's. At the time Jim was sitting up and so I listened with a stethoscope while he was in that position and after twenty five or so beats I heard just one PVC's. I repeated listening in that position once again with the same results. I then asked him to lie on his back while I listened to his heart. Again and again I got the same results. I told Jim that I was sorry he even knew about his skips – that they were rather infrequent and clinically insignificant. I told him about the number of beats I heard before I detected a skip and he was amazed to the point of disbelief because they had always been a lot more frequent than that. I explained that while they may have been more frequent at one time they certainly were not now. During his next visit to my office he told me that he had seen his family medical doctor since our last meeting and that he stood before him with his mouth agape in almost disbelief that the PVC's were gone!

"How can that be?" Jim asked. I explained that during his monthly treatments one of the acupuncture points stimulated was Bladder 15 located at the fifth thoracic vertebra and that it is directly associated with the heart. I reminded him that the meridians are connected with one another and stimulating that particular point brought energy to it allowing the body to heal the heart condition. The body heals itself.

After Bob Holt left his office Tom began reflecting upon other remarkable incidents that he had had using acupuncture. He decided that probably the case of sciatic neuralgia was the most dramatic in terms of recovery that he had seen. He remembered the incident but not the name of the patient. The patient was the mother of a woman who called the office one day asking if I could see her mother preferably on that day. I came to the phone to talk with her and assure her that I would make time for her mother.

"Is it all right if she comes in her pajamas?" she asked. And then added that she was going to have to arrange for an ambulance to bring her because she could barely move due to the pain. She had been in bed for two solid weeks with acute sciatic pain.

"She's that acute?" I asked.

"Yes, she has been in awful pain." Tom had a better idea to make a house call and found out that they didn't live too far from his office. So, he made arrangements to see her later that day.

"What have you been doing for it?" Tom asked the mother when he arrived.

"The doctor told me to use a heating pad and stay in bed. He also prescribed some pain pills that don't seem to help. A heating pad for two weeks, thought Tom. My God, it's no wonder she has such spasm in her muscles. She was able to roll over onto one side allowing Tom an opportunity to insert needles into her lower back. During the twenty minutes the needles were left in place he answered some questions from the patient as well as her daughter and also advised her to discontinue the heating pad immediately and substitute it with ice packs. He said an ice pack should remain on her low back for about twenty minutes at a time and that it is all right to lie directly on it if you wish. He asked her to repeat this cryotherapy at least three or four times before he returned tomorrow for a second acupuncture treatment.

"But my medical doctor told me to use the heating pad," she said.

"Heat is a very common mistake in the treatment of acute cases," I replied. "Trust me on this. You need to break up that severe muscle spasm with ice. Much of the muscle spasm was caused by too much heat." She agreed to follow his suggestions. The next day when Tom arrived at their house he was pleasantly surprised to see his patient out of bed and sitting in a lounge chair next to it. The third and last day of treatment, she walked into Tom's office and he never saw her again. The pleasure that Tom got from seeing her respond so dramatically was almost orgasmic. Tom had had other cases of patients with severe muscle spasms. He recalled a time when two men were carrying another into his office on an ironing board. The 'stiff' on the ironing board had slept the entire night with the heating pad on and to make matters worse had even slept on it. You never want to lie on top of a heating pad when it's on because hot spots develop easily and can cause a nasty burn. Many in the medical profession just don't seem to understand the physiology behind acute muscle spasm. Heat causes the blood vessels to expand to a point where they begin to leak plasma into the surrounding tissues. The innate reaction is for the body to contract the musculature in an attempt to prevent the loss of fluid from the blood. When muscles contract they squeeze the blood vessels down preventing them from bringing a sufficient supply of oxygen to the area and again the natural defensive response is for the muscles to contract even further. It is a vicious cycle that, if not interrupted, can produce severe pain and poor mobility. Although ice does indeed have a tendency to contract blood vessels, muscles etc. the fact that it slows everything down overshadows any effect from contraction.

On the drive home many suspicious thoughts about Bob Holt's visit entered his mind. Does he have an ulterior motive? Why did he choose me above all the other chiropractors in town? He lived closer to several other chiropractors but chose to come to me. Did Shane, Bailey and White put him up to this, he wondered. Are they trying to get something else on me? Was he placed here as a spy? Maybe I'm blowing this out of proportion and he really is a nice guy seeking some help. I'll check around to see if he really does have congestive heart disease. After all not many ,if any, of the other chiropractors practice acupuncture. I would be within my legal right to refuse to treat him. If I did treat him, though, I'd be able to kind of keep my eye on him and see if he had things on his mind other than his congestive heart disease. Tom's concentration was so focused that he just sat there at an intersection after the traffic light had turned green – much to the displeasure of a red neck in a utility 4x4 truck behind him with a hand glued to its horn. C'mon move it you ole bastard, he yelled. Tom shook his head as if coming out of a daze and promptly pushed down on the accelerator and moved out regretting that he didn't give the rude guy a 'finger'.

"What kept you so long today?" June asked when he entered the kitchen door.

"I was delayed with a new patient. And you'll never guess who it is."

"Is it Judge O'Malley?"

"No but you're on the right track. It's Bob Holt, the guy who sued me for three million bucks and now wants me to help him with his congestive heart condition."

"Did he mention anything about the trial?"

"Not a word, nor did I. I kept it strictly on the professional side. But it sure gave me cause to wonder on the way home. I don't know whether this thing is on the up and up or if he and his lawyers are trying to nail me with something. What do you think?"

"Well I think that if you refused to treat him he might consider that an admission that you were guilty of his wife's death, but if you continue in your professional manner as if nothing had occurred in the past he's apt to reconsider his opinion altogether. I think you should continue and as you indicated it'll keep you in fairly close contact with the man to see if he's genuine about his heart condition or still dreaming of three million."

"I think you're right – as usual – I'll do the best that I can for him. How is it that I can get myself all worked up over things and in a five or ten minute conversation with you everything seems clear and right?"

"It's a gift."

Saturday is not a day off for Tom Clayton. He tries to get away from the office by noon or shortly thereafter but it's usually three of four o'clock before he can leave. This of course effectively cuts his weekends in half. But he doesn't mind because he loves his work and long hours 'go with the territory'. It's truly a necessity to be available on Saturdays to serve persons who find it difficult, if not impossible, to get to his office during the week because of their job responsibilities. And June, bless her heart, has never complained. Even before she married Tom she knew what to expect as a wife of a doctor. She has even learned to cope with an occasional interruption at home when Tom was called out for a house call. Their income is sufficient to afford a membership in a country club near by affording June plenty of opportunities to keep occupied playing tennis, golf, bridge and the triple 'L' club or Ladies Lucidity League. It's not really a club at all since it lacks a charter, bylaws etc. but rather its Tom's sarcastic rendition of women gathering for gossip.

It was a Saturday morning when Barbara, his nurse, receptionist and trusted confidant, caught him in the hallway between treatment rooms to let Tom know that Mrs. Charlotte K.... wishes to speak with him on the telephone.

"Please tell her that I'm in the middle of something right now and that I'll return her call the first chance I get." Barbara nodded and went back to the phone. Charlotte and Jay K.... had been patients for about two years, kept their appointments, were always on time and paid their bills promptly. Tom's favorite kind of patient. Charlotte had always worked at a sedentary type of job before she decided to try retailing. That infatuation soon left as she found that long hours on her feet were causing a chronic and annoying pain in her left foot. It was a genuine pain as opposed to simple soreness or tiredness. Examination and comparison of both feet revealed a subluxated bone in her left foot which was pronounced enough to be noticeable with a naked eye. Pronounced and stubborn. It took Tom three visits before he felt the bone slide back into place. The pain she was experiencing disappeared almost immediately. When Charlotte became pregnant, not from any of Tom's treatment mind you, he treated her for occasional back pain with chiropractic adjustments in conjunction with acupuncture. They became fast friends.

Jay sought help to break his smoking habit. He was smoking a pack to a pack and a half of cigarettes daily. He tried to 'kick the habit' several times in the past only to succumb to an overpowering desire to have a cigarette. Tom had smoked in the past and remembered what a compelling urge it was to smoke. Some patients turned to hypnotism which was helpful but seemed to dampen the urge for only three of four months. Most who had tried it did not return for further treatments because they considered the cost prohibitive. At that time a hypnotic session was running between eighty five and one hundred dollars each. Tom's packaged program met this challenge. He charged $100.00 due and payable at the time of the first visit which entitled an individual to a total of five treatments if needed. If more than five treatments might be required additional ones would cost $20.00 each. If the patient required only one or two treatments there was no refund from the original $100.00. This program was met with enthusiasm by his patients since it was quite affordable and assured their cooperation in keeping appointments since they were prepaid. With every new patient trying to stop smoking Tom cautioned him/her to be absolutely determined they wanted to quit smoking and that an attitude of "okay, Charlie, show me" was destined for failure. A positive attitude and exercise of some will power was absolutely essential to the success of any non smoking program. While the acupuncture needles are in place for twenty minutes the patient is requested to frequently repeat to him/herself

"I am becoming a non smoker," which is a positive reinforcement whereas mantras such as I'll never smoke again, I'm not going to smoke and the like are negative thoughts. Patients are also encouraged to establish short and attainable goals toward their deserved abstinence. For example: Let's see if you can go a half hour without smoking. I've gone a half hour let's see if I can go another half hour. Once that's accomplished you would set a goal for one more hour. And so it would go until, say, lunch time, after which you would again shorten the goal by saying I've gone a half a day let's see if I can go another half a day. Etc. until goals no longer become necessary because you are now a NON SMOKER!! After just three treatments Jay had completely lost the urge to smoke and hasn't touched a cigarette in twenty some odd years much to his credit.

"Hi Charlotte. This is Tom Clayton returning your call. Is that child you're carrying causing some back pain again?"

"No my back is fine. That child is late. I'm two weeks overdue. Are there some points you can needle that'll help me drop this kid?"

"As a matter of fact, there are. Why don't you come in any time after 1:00 today and we'll see what we can do." The rest is history of course. She did come to the office later that day, got treated and delivered a beautiful baby girl the following day. From that point on Dr. Clayton could never do anything wrong in the eyes of Charlotte K….- he walks on water.

Chapter 7

"Here Barbara, doc might be interested in this article." It was a copy of East & West Magazine opened to an article about electrical stimulation.

"Thank you Mr. Hadley. I'm certain the doctor will be interested. I'll put it on his desk so that he'll be sure to see it. He's in with your mother now and she should be out shortly." Hadley nodded and picked up another magazine off the rack and sat down.

Later after June and Tom had eaten dinner and cleaned up the kitchen they settled into the den. June wanted to watch 'The Wheel of Fortune' on the television and Tom picked up the magazine that Chris Hadley had left. At first glance he noticed a picture of an electrical stimulation instrument that looked like a familiar TENS unit. TENS is an acronym for transcutaneous electrical nerve stimulator and they are in common use for musculoskeletal pain control. Electrical stimulation for medical purposes predates the last century and was highly successful for a variety of conditions. Successful, that is until charlatans began flooding the market with virtually empty boxes with dials and gauges that did nothing. These charlatans effectively destroyed the use of electricity in medicine for decades and it wasn't until the beginning of the twentieth century that it began to gain recognition and trust again. Electrical stimulation helps to break up muscle spasm, increases blood flow to an injured area bringing fresh oxygen and nutrients needed for healing and encourages lymph and venous drainage of waste materials from the area. These instruments are available as portable units that can be hooked onto a belt or carried in a pocket. Doctors loan, lease and sell these instruments directly to their patients. The stimulating current supplied by a battery is delivered by means of self- adhesive electrodes strategically placed to pass current through the injured area. A major draw back in their application is that they are effective only when the unit is on. When not in use, pain usually returns.

But the instrument described in the East & West magazine is not just another TENS unit. The article relates to a microamperage electrical stimulator called the Alpha Stim. TENS units are all designed to deliver milliamperage current which is defined as a thousandth of an ampere whereas microamperage stimulators are defined in millionths of an ampere. Although that makes microamperage current a thousand times less than milliamperes some might say it is a thousand times more effective from a physiological standpoint. The body has a natural flow of bioelectrical current throughout except where there is a blockage in the form of an injury. Milliamperage current, as in TENS instruments simply moves around an area of injury but microamperage current passes directly through. In effect, then, microamperage stimulators re-establish the normal bioelectric flow whereas milliamperage stimulators do not. And once normal bioelectric flow is established the body is better able to heal itself and pain is relieved permanently even after the instrument is shut off. It's easy to question how such a mild current is able to penetrate the body deep enough to accomplish any healing at all but if you imagine a long tube filled with ping pong balls and what would happen if you introduced one more ping pong ball at either end you have a pretty good idea of the concept involved.

With microamperage instruments battery generated electrical current is delivered to patients by means of probes, self adhesive pads and clips that fasten to ear lobes. Probe application is quite specific and lends itself to stimulation of acupuncture points very nicely. Pad electrodes cover a much broader area and can be situated in such a manner as to place a pain area in between two or four of them. Ear clip electrodes are unique in that current flows across the skull at the level of the hypothalamus which is that portion of the brain that regulates so many vital and basic body functions.

Tom read the entire article with growing intensity. His first question was how effective would microamperage electrical stimulation be as a substitute for needles in treating someone with acupuncture. Most patients really don't care for needles of any kind – thin or not. Some people are actually afraid of them. Two of Tom's patients in the past actually began going into shock during an acupuncture treatment. Admittedly two patients in fifteen or twenty years of practice is not a significant percentage but nonetheless apprehension must be present in a large number of patients that don't show signs of going into shock. He decided to call Dr. Dan Kirsch who was noted in the article as the developer and CEO of a company marketing the Alpha Stim. Tom was quite anxious to learn the cost of these instruments because he knew the stationary models sold for about $10,000.00 a piece. To outfit his four treatment rooms with one of those would cost about $40,000.00 a cost out of the question at least for now.

"Good morning Barbara. Anyone here yet?"

"Mr. Holt is in room one and you have a new patient coming in for a consultation in a half an hour."

"Thank you. Do me a favor, please, and call Dr. Kirsch at this number," handing Barbara a slip of paper with the number written upon it, "and ask him if it would be convenient for me to call him around noon to discuss the Alpha Stim instrument."

"Of course." And with that Tom entered room one.

"Good morning Mr. Holt."

"Good morning doctor." After exchanging pleasantries Tom asked him to lie upon his stomach and then inserted several acupuncture needles into association points along the spine making certain he didn't overlook Bladder 15 located at the 5th vertebra in the back below the seven cervical vertebrae which is associated directly with the heart.

"Have you had any blood work done, Mr. Holt?"

"Oh yes, several times."

"Would you know what your homocysteine count is?"

"Homo sis teen? Never heard of it."

"It's a protein formed by the metabolism of another protein called methionine. Normal levels go as high as 15 micromoles per liter but are elevated beyond that in arthritis, osteoporosis, Alzheimer's disease, stroke and heart disease. It is a far better indicator of heart disease than cholesterol ever was. The idea that high levels of cholesterol cause heart attacks, in my opinion, is a fraudulent myth perpetrated and perpetuated by the pharmaceutical companies in order to sell more Statin drugs to lower it. Several facts belie this contention: First, 60% of the people who suffer a heart attack have normal cholesterol. I don't know what level was used as a standard as the pharmaceutical industry keeps lowering it. In the past, I have worked with laboratories that considered cholesterol levels to be normal between 215 and 300 mg./dl to be normal. Now they are telling us that 200 mg./dl is too high. Second, believe it or not, most people with high cholesterol don't have heart diseases. Third, 50% of those who suffered a heart attack didn't have any of the risk factors such as obesity, high blood pressure, smoking and genetic factors. Fourth, Eskimos have a diet very rich in cholesterol and yet they experience far less heart disease than we in America. Admittedly their diet is quite high in HDL, the good cholesterol, and low in LDL, the bad cholesterol. Fifth, a ten year study conducted by the Swiss involving 475 females and 437 males showed that there was no correlation whatsoever between the dietary intake of cholesterol and blood levels of it. This was reported in the American Journal of Medicine. Sixth, approximately 420 people die every day due to a deficiency of magnesium. That's over 150,000 people a year!

As you might expect there is a flip side to the cholesterol story. There is such a thing as too little cholesterol as well. Cholesterol is vital to our very existence so much so that Mother Nature saw to it that our bodies make it. The liver produces between 1500 and 1800 mg. every day. By comparison our dietary intake is only about 400 mg. per day. Cholesterol is a part of every cell, a constituent of many hormones, a major part of bile salts for digestion, makes vitamin D as well as steroid hormones and is critical to nerve function. A plethora of independent studies involving some 79,000 subjects have clearly demonstrated tat low levels of cholesterol, levels below 160 mg./dl, can cause heart attacks. In fact the risk is considerably higher than the risk with higher cholesterol. We mentioned that cholesterol is needed to make vitamin D which in turn is necessary for the adequate absorption of calcium. Therefore, if cholesterol is deficient poor calcium absorption could lead to osteoporosis. We also noted that cholesterol is required for proper nerve function in that it forms a substance called acetylcholine that allows for the propagation of nerve impulses. Low levels of cholesterol, then, could provide a link to such neurological diseases as Alzheimer's, Parkinson's and ALS. ALS is amyotrophic lateral sclerosis better known as Lou Gehrig's disease. Since statin drugs as well as insecticides, pesticides etc. are know to decrease cholesterol it is possible that once again MAN in his infinite stupidity is creating more problems than he is solving."

"I had no idea," Bob Holt said, "Why don't they tell you things like this?"

"Simply because they don't want you to know about it. Their interest is in selling more statin drugs."

"What about the government? Why doesn't the FDA intercede?

"In my opinion, Mr. Holt, the Food and Drug Administration's main purpose is to protect the profits of the pharmaceutical industry. Sixty percent of its employees were formerly employed by pharmaceutical companies. Look how long they protected Merck's profits while Vioxx killed over 100,000 people. Both the FDA and Merck knew the dangers of Vioxx before it was even marketed. It is certainly true that cholesterol is a part of the atherosclerotic plague that forms a clot but why pick on cholesterol. There are other elements involved such as fibrin, lipids, platelets and even calcium. As a matter of fact fibrin arrives at the scene before cholesterol. You may not realize, Mr. Holt, that our bodies make cholesterol – quite a bit of it every day. It's a component of every cell in our body and we each have about seventy five trillion of them, it's necessary for the production of vitamin D, is a component of bile salts for digestion purposes and is an important part of nerve function. Finally, bear in mind that when blood is drawn for a cholesterol study it is usually taken from a vein in the bend of an elbow. But we never see atherosclerosis occurring in a vein. It's always in an artery. So there must be a difference between a vein and an artery. And indeed there is. An artery has an additional muscle layer not found in veins and it is this muscle layer that is attacked and where plague builds up forming a clot."

"Well, if cholesterol is not the cause of heart disease, what is?"

"It's the damage to the muscle layer I just mentioned that provides a focal point for the accumulation of blood elements and eventual build up of plague producing a clot. A prevalent cause of damage to arterial walls is from nasty things called free radicals which are oxygen molecules that lack an electron and in search of electrons they attack normal tissue such as the interior wall of arteries. Free radicals are formed during normal metabolic processes and it has been estimated that we form about ten thousand of them every day. Other things that damage arterial walls include chlorine, trans fats, hydrogenated oils, homogenized dairy products and homocysteine.

"Are you still concerned about your cholesterol level Mr. Holt?"

"Yes, I'd really like to get it down below 260."

"If so, there are several alternative approaches in lieu of toxic drugs that are open to you. (Appendix 'A'). Red Yeast Rice available in health food stores has been effective for many people. It should be approached with caution , however, since it has the same molecular structure as the statin drugs. Therefore, I'm not recommending it in your case. One thing I strongly recommend, though, is that you discard any and all microwaves that you might own. They are notorious for raising cholesterol levels."

"Really," said Bob Holt with an amazed look on his face.

"Really," answered Tom. "Even if you were not interested in lowering your cholesterol microwaves are still bad for us. They alter the molecular makeup of food and cause cancer. The microwave was invented by the Nazis but thoroughly researched by the Russians. They are the ones that learned how food was altered in microwave ovens and caused cancer. I don't know about today but there was a time when you couldn't buy a microwave in Russia – they were outlawed. You and your wife…oh I forgot. I am terribly sorry Mr. Holt."

"That's okay, doctor, I'm pretty well over that by now. I guess it's high time anyway to apologize for bringing those charges against you. I wasn't in it for the money I was simply venting my anger and hurt and you happened to be my choice. I faired fairly well as a stock broker, the house and automobiles are all free and clear and both daughters are out of the nest and doing quite well. So, please go on with what you started."

"I was about to tell you of a test that you can run in your own home that illustrates how microwaves alter things. Purchase some seeds and place them into two pots. Water one pot with ordinary tap water and the other with water that has been nuked in your microwave oven. The seeds watered with nuked water will never germinate! If it can alter water like that, think what it might do to your foodstuffs. If you are not currently supplementing your diet with some Omega 3 oils I would recommend that you do so. They can be very helpful in lowering cholesterol also. If after a few months your cholesterol is still elevated beyond your desire we can try other approaches all of which are easy on your wallet.

Policosonol made from the same plant from which we get cane sugar increases HDL (high density lipoprotein) and lowers LDL. It, too can be purchased in health food stores. Tocotrienols which are a part of the vitamin E complex have also been helpful. Arjuna, a commercial product, in addition to decreasing the pain of angina, preventing ischemia and improving congestive heart disease also decreases LDL. Lecithin, which is Greek for egg yolk, aids in liquefying cholesterol which normally melts at 145 degrees centigrade or 293 degrees Fahrenheit.

To help further prevent heart disease there are some measures that might prove to be helpful to you. (Appendix 'B') Number one would be to take a complete multi vitamin/mineral supplement daily. One that was also loaded with antioxidants to combat free radicals. Six thousand studies have shown that vitamin E can reduce the risk of heart attacks by 50%. Stepping up the consumption of magnesium, which is a natural muscle relaxant, and drastically reducing your sugar consumption both help to lower blood pressure. Natural blood thinners that help to lower blood pressure include omega 3 oils, magnesium, vitamin E preferably with tocotrienols, garlic, policosonol and bromelain from pineapple juice."

"Thank you, this has been most informative. I'll get those supplements on the way home."

"You're welcome. I hope you might be able to draw something useful from our discussion." Tom left the room, informed Barbara when Mr. Holt's needles should be removed and entered the next treatment room.

"Hello Mrs. Mead. I'm doctor Clayton. How may we be of help?"

"I've been diagnosed with uterine cancer and they want to give me chemotherapy. And not only do I not want it, I won't take it. A neighbor of mine told me about your conservative approaches to health and I'm wondering if you might be able to help me."

"Let me tell you what I know and think about cancer and then let you decide if you feel that we might be of some help to you. I know, for example, without any further discussion or conducting any type of examination that your body was exposed to some toxin that produced the cancerous tumor and that your body is probably quite acidic in nature. I am certain of this because a biologic researcher by the name of Dr. Otto Wallberg won a Nobel Prize for discovering that cancer cells and viruses cannot exist in an alkaline environment. So the trick is to make our bodies as alkaline as possible. As far as the cause of your cancer is concerned it is after the fact but we are all exposed to a multitude of toxic chemicals every day many of which are carcinogenic. Take pesticides for example. Of the sixty four of them in common use today sixteen have been proven to cause cancer, 24 can cause brain damage and forty four create hormonal variations. Nice, huh? Your immediate concern, of course, is to get rid of the tumor you have and prevent it from spreading or metastasizing to other organs. But first let me give you some effective things you can do to prevent cancer from redeveloping. These are things I would most assuredly do and I recommend you discuss them with your healthcare professional. Certainly I would want to avoid as many toxins as I could. We'll give you a partial list of some of the more common ones found in products used everyday before you leave today. (Appendix 'C'). We should all be eating as many organically grown foods as possible to avoid the use of insecticides, pesticides etc. that are very harmful to us. I realize the cost of organic foods is higher than other foods but if more people would demand organically grown products the price would come down to a more realistic level. All prescription and nonprescription drugs are toxic – even such common products as laxatives and Alka Seltzer. We don't need them. There are always alternative approaches to these harmful substances that do nothing but put money into the pockets of the manufacturers. Reactions to prescription drugs currently are the fourth leading cause of deaths in the country. They also represent the fourth most common reason for going to a hospital. We should all be eating more alkaline ash foods than acid ash ones. (Appendices "D' & 'E'). Alkaline ash foods should comprise at least seventy five percent of our diets. This might deserve further explanation. The body simply does not like acid. The only place it wants it is in the stomach to help with the digestion of protein and to aid the absorption of calcium. We rid ourselves of acid in two basic ways. When we exhale we are getting rid of carbonic acid in the form of carbon dioxide. Another mechanism is known as the alkaline reserve which counteracts acids by forming neutral salts with them which are easily expelled by the body. Everything else is alkaline. Blood is alkaline. Lymph is alkaline. Digestive enzymes and hormones are also. After our foods are digested a residue or ash remains and this ash will be either acid or alkaline. As I mentioned earlier we should eat more alkaline ash foods than acid ash ones and Barbara will give you a list of example of both that you can use as a guide for diet purposes. Don't be fooled by some of the foods you see listed. For example we all know that grapefruit is quite acid. It might register three or four on a litmus chart but the ash that is left is very alkaline and would register well above the neutral seven on a litmus chart, maybe as high as nine. Refined carbohydrates should be drastically curtailed from our diets. They are made from refined flours and sugars and quickly turn to glucose in the body. Unfortunately they are represented by everything that tastes so good – pies, cakes, cookies, donuts and all kinds of tasty snacks. Complex carbohydrates, on the other hand, are good for us. These include potatoes, beans, lentils and grains that are not absorbed as readily as the simple carbohydrates. Sugar should all but be eliminated from our diets. Unfortunately, there are hidden sugars in all kinds of grocery products that we buy. (Appendices 'F', 'G' & 'H'). Six ounces of Ginger Ale contains approximately five teaspoons of sugar. A four ounce piece of iced chocolate cake has ten teaspoons of sugar in it. Four ounces of hard candy is equivalent to ten Hershey bars and contains about 20 teaspoons of sugar. Nabisco's 100% bran is almost twenty percent sugar. The list goes on and on – check your labels and learn how often sugar appears!! Finally, you might consider doing what my wife and I do on a daily basis. We drink a capful – not a cupful – of hydrogen peroxide in six or eight ounces of water or juice. This is ordinary 3% inexpensive hydrogen peroxide you can purchase at any drug store. Oxygenating the body in this fashion helps to make it alkaline and unfriendly to cancer cells and viruses.

Before we talk about some alternative treatments for cancer there are a couple of things you should learn about cancer cells themselves. First, they are dissimilar cells to that of the organ affected. That is to say a cancerous tumor of say, the uterus, is not made up of all uterine cells. These cancer cells, unlike normal ones, can metabolize or use glucose without the presence of oxygen. Also in utilizing glucose cancer cells form lactic acid which in turn is processed by the liver to form, of all things, more glucose. This sets up a vicious cycle and explains how and why cancer cells spread or metastasize so rapidly taking over tissues, organs and often lives. There is good news, however. There are products available to break up this vicious cycle and destroy cancerous tumors. The first one called hydrazine sulfate is designed to prevent the liver from processing lactic acid formed by the cancer cells. It has been thoroughly researched by Dr. Joseph Gold of the Cancer Research Institute of Syracuse University. Were I you, I would get on that medication immediately and if you become a patient of ours, I would certainly prescribe it. The second product is called Avemar and acts to inhibit cancer cells from utilizing glucose so it should be taken along with hydrazine sulfate. Both of these products, then, effectively break up the vicious cycle we talked about. Hydrazine sulfate is very inexpensive but Avemar costs a little more, but far less than chemotherapy, because it is made from a special fermented wheat grown in Hungary.

Alternative cures are not new, Mrs. Mead. There have been many of them in the past. We just don't hear of them because they all were widely discredited by a conglomerate interested in furthering the sales of expensive profit laden patented drugs. This conglomerate includes the Food and Drug Administration, American Medical Association, National Cancer Institute, American Cancer Society and the pharmaceutical industry as a whole. I'll mention just a few and I'm sure you will be pleasantly surprised to learn what's out there for you:

Dr. Harry Hoxsey treated 10,000 patients with a yellow compound and red salve along with an internal tonic with an 80% cure rate. Chemotherapy, radiation and surgery combined can't even approach that record with their puny 3% cure rate.

Dr. William Koch treated cancer patients for thirty years with a compound called glyoxylide until the FDA closed him down.

Dr. Royal Rife developed a microscope under which bacteria and viruses could be seen. That's commonplace today but this was back in the nineteen twenties. He also developed a ray tube that selectively killed cancer cells and left normal cells untouched. Think of that way back in the twenties and cancer still on the increase. Shameful. When he refused to sell both the microscope and ray tube to the AMA all doctors were informed by the them that they would have their license taken away if caught using either instrument. Free enterprise at work.

Dr. Andrew Ivy battled with the AMA and NCI over the use of kreibiozen as a treatment for cancer. He tried in vain to get them to test the product. They not only refused they published lies about the product and discredited Dr. Ivy mercilessly.

In Mexico Dr. Curt Donsbach treated cancer patients with DMSO, which is dimethylsulfoxide, along with hydrogen peroxide with fantastic results. Other Mexican hospitals used hydrogen peroxide and ozone also with virtually 100% success. These procedures are now available in the United States although not sanctioned by orthodox medicine.

Dr. Gasten Naessen developed a microscope capable of viewing all blood elements. He developed a chemical he called 714-X which also is highly successful in treating cancer.

I have already mention Dr. Joseph Gold of the Syracuse Cancer Research Institute and the discovery that hydrazine sulfate proved successful in treating cancer. The AMA and NCI finally agreed to test his product but did so under false pretenses. Patients who take hydrazine sulfate must not take any barbiturates, tranquillizers, pain killing drugs or alcohol. Everyone of the subjects in the bogus AMA study was in violation of these premises so they reported that hydrazine sulfate was worthless. Another piece of wool pulled over our eyes.

More recent treatments include the following:

The American Journal of Preventive Medicine reported that increasing vitamin D by 1000 – 2000 International Units per day reduces the risk of colon cancer by 50%.

Fucoidan, marketed as Modifilian is found in brown seaweed. It causes cancer cells to self-destruct a process called apoptosis.

AHCC or Active Hexose Correlated Compound is a tremendous immune system booster. It can increase our killer cells by 300% so that the body is better able to destroy any cancer cells. It is produced from the shiitake mushroom and works best in conjunction with Modifilian just mentioned.

Graviola is an extract from the graviola tree. Along with seven other immune boosting herbs it is marketed under the trade name N-Tense. This product seeks out and destroys cancer cells. A pharmaceutical company spent seven years trying to duplicate this extract synthetically and sell a patented drug for profit. When they failed, they buried the research material from public use. A conscientious employee finally divulged the clandestine action and the product finally became available to the public. We mentioned Avemar earlier and its ability to cut off the energy supply to cancer cells.

I hope all this has been of some help to you Mrs. Mead."

"Indeed it has. During your discourse I decided that I should like to become one of your patients."

"That's fine, Mrs. Mead, please pick up those lists we talked about from Barbara on the way out and ask her to set up another appointment as soon as possible so that we can start getting you back to normal."

After talking with Dr. Kirsch Tom decided to buy three portable Alpha Stim instruments. He began using them in three of his four treatment rooms in place of acupuncture needles and found his patients willing to cooperate. It certainly made life easier for Barbara who was used to autoclaving (sterilizing) several batches of needles every day. Now the number of batches has been reduced she has more time to devote to her many other duties. Patient acceptance of the Alpha Stim treatments was not universal however. There was a small group of five patients being treated for Benign Essential Blepharospasm, or BEB. Essential used in the medical sense means 'of unknown origin' or cause. Blepharospasm refers to spasm of the eyelids. Tom was introduced to this disease from one of his patients who suffered from it but was being treated by Tom for other conditions. It was during one of her visits that she outspokenly suggested that he attend one of their support group meetings. Tom agreed as he was quite anxious to learn more about this strange disease. Before the scheduled day of their meeting, Tom had already decided to offer acupuncture treatments in his office free of charge to volunteers in an effort to learn if acupuncture was a viable treatment for BEB. He treated each volunteer at least twice a week and added electrical current to select needles. Blepharospasm fortunately is not very widely spread affecting some 50,000 people. Those that are affected, however, experience some awful moments. It's a terrible thing to witness when an afflicted patient has a spasmodic attack. Their eyes are spontaneously clamped shut and cannot be opened even by prying. It's easy for one to imagine the perils associated with driving a car, bicycle or other means of transportation. These victims, then, are necessarily very limited in their activities at work, out of doors and even at home. During a spasm attack the victim simply 'waits it out' for the spasm to subside so that they can resume normal activities. The Alpha Stim by itself was not particularly effective on any of the patients. Each seemed to require the additional electrical stimulation provided with acupuncture needles. As a matter of interest, three of the five patients responded very well with two experiencing complete cures and one improved significantly over the length of the study. A fourth patient had had nerves removed from the areas selected for acupuncture treatments. The fifth patient had dropped out of the study after just one or two treatments. The study was published in the American Journal of Acupuncture and to date remains the only study of its kind to the best of Tom's knowledge.

Chapter 8

The reception room was simply jammed. Not with patients but with chairs. Barbara had rented some folding chairs and she and Tom were setting up the reception room for an evening seminar for his patients. Some chairs were even set up in the entranceway to a hallway leading to treatment rooms as they were expecting a pretty good turn out judging from comments they heard during the week. On a corner table in the back of the room sat two urns – one containing coffee and the other hot water for tea drinkers. For those not wanting to drink any caffeine after dinner some chilled Spicy Hot V8 juice was available. Two dishes of assorted nuts were available as substitutes for the customary sugar laden cookies or cakes. On each chair they placed a small pad of paper and a Bic pen for those wishing to make notes along with three handouts: Toxic Pollutants To Avoid; Alkaline Ash Foods; and Acid Ash Foods. When patients started arriving both Tom and Barbara wondered if there was going to be enough room for all of them. Luck was on their side and all patients were able to find a chair. Tom thought there must have been close to thirty people there and he saw a few unfamiliar faces. Good, he thought, maybe we can get some new patients from this seminar. There were friends and neighbors of existing patients who might become impressed with what they saw and learned this evening. At 7:00 P.M. on the nose Tom stood before those assembled and greeted them warmly thanking them for taking the time to attend..

"Tonight ladies and gentlemen by your popular choice we'll be discussing the many toxins to which we are exposed everyday and that are taking their toll with our health. I sincerely hope that you will find the time well spent and will be able to take away something of benefit to your health."

"Communicable diseases," he began, "such as measles, scarlet fever and the like are pretty much under control thanks in part to improved sanitation and effective antibiotics. Chronic degenerative diseases, however, are not and in fact most, if not all, are on the increase. We catch colds, the flu and other communicable diseases but we don't catch arthritis, cancer, osteoporosis, Alzheimer's or a myriad of other degenerative diseases. From where do they come? They come from toxins that we ingest, inhale, inject and absorb into our bodies everyday. The Environmental Protection Agency states that of the 70,000 chemicals used commercially 65,000 are potentially dangerous. The Environmental Defense Group has said that of the four billion pounds of toxic chemicals released every year that 72 million of them are known carcinogens. The World Health Organization tells us that two million people die every year from air pollution. Scary isn't it? Surprisingly we are subjected to five times more toxins in our homes than we are out of doors. That may be hard for you to believe, but check the labels of products you use in your home. You might see diethanolamine listed in your shampoo or hair conditioner. You might also find it listed on your body lotion or even one of your cosmetics. Diethanolamine has been proven to cause cancer! Do you use air fresheners? Most of them contain glycol esters and terpenes which combine with ozone in the air to form formaldehyde. That's embalming fluid! You might also notice in your shampoos, toothpastes and soaps an ingredient called propylene glycol which happens to be the main ingredient of antifreeze for your automobiles. This chemical causes kidney and liver damage, produces nausea, vomiting and deep depression. Maybe you'll see sodium lauryl sulfate listed in the same products. This chemical is so strong that it is used to clean grease off the floors in auto garages. One teaspoon will kill you! It also affects the liver, heart and lungs by altering genetic cell structure causing cancer. Yes, toxins are all around us: dry cleaning fluids, mothballs, toilet bowl cleaners and even ink toners in your computer printer and fax machines. Manufacturers are killing us in the interest of greater profits for themselves. Most products now carry an 800 number you can call if you have questions or comments about their product.

A couple of household items deserve special attention. The first one we'll talk about is fluorine. Regardless of what you have been led to believe fluorine is a poison worse than lead. It destroys the immune system and causes asthma, thyroid conditions and cancer. It also destroys collagen leading to osteoporosis or arthritis or both.   It makes us fatter and increases the absorption of aluminum which many   believe is a strong link to Alzheimer's disease. It causes calcification of the pineal gland which is linked to early puberty in females and bone cancer in males. Now, there's a combination for you. Fluorine is a by-product in the production of aluminum and is sold as an insecticide and rat poison. And, believe it or not, it does NOT prevent tooth decay!! A very extensive Swiss study proved that there is no validity to the claim that fluorine prevents tooth decay. Dr. Dean, the father of fluorine, testified under oath that no research existed to verify the claim that fluorine prevented tooth decay. Nevertheless it is still found in some municipal drinking water, mouth washes, bottled water products and of course toothpastes. Yes, you have a question, Mrs. Marley?"

"Why haven't we heard about this from our dentists or read about it in newspapers?"

"This hasn't been widely publicized probably to avoid costly class action law suits. As you now know from what we've discussed that a multitude of industries could be named in such a law suit.

"Does that answer your question okay, Mrs. Marley?"

"Yes it does, thank you."

"T he other common ingredient that needs special attention is soy which according to Dr. William Campbell Douglass is closely linked to indigestion, allergies, impotency, thyroid disease, loss of mentality and finally cancer. It DOES NOT, as has been publicized, lower cholesterol or reduce hot flushes. Several European countries have abandoned its use but here in the United States it is still a constituent of some 60% of our grocery products. Soy is an animal feed that is loaded with female hormones that cause early puberty in females and homosexuality in males. Now if you will refer to the handout 'Toxic Pollutants to Avoid' we'll go over a few of the common ones to which we are exposed. The first one listed there is aspartame. It is marketed as Nutrasweet, Equal or Spoonful but is also found in some five hundred other products. Incidentally, Splenda is no better as an artificial sweetener. Aspartame use has shown to cause an increase in the incidence of multiple sclerosis and lupus. It produces a craving for simple refined carbohydrates assuring a weight gain from continued use. Some symptoms to look for, if you are a user, would be fibromyalgia, muscle spasms, shooting pains, leg cramps or numbness, vertigo, headaches, tinnitus or ringing in the ears, joint pains, blurred vision and memory loss. That pretty well covers the water front, doesn't it? With such a broad list of symptoms, I should think aspartame would be a good product to avoid.

The next is chlorine. It, like fluorine, is a poison. We can ingest it from municipal water supplies and absorb it through our skin while swimming in a chlorinated pool. Chlorine scars interior walls of arteries leading to atherosclerotic plaguing and possible heart attack.

We have already talked about diethanolamine. Diethylstilbesterol is another poison that speeds sexual maturity in females and is found as a residual in 85% of all meat products. Next on the list is fluorine which we have also covered in some detail. Glycol esters, remember, form formaldehyde by combining with ozone in the air and are frequent ingredients of aerosols. Hexachlorophene is a poison to prevent bacterial growth but is still found in many cosmetics, soaps and detergents.

High fructose corn syrup is getting to be an ubiquitous ingredient in our food products. You can see it listed in soft drinks, jellies and jams, breakfast cereals and almost any product that contains sweeteners of any kind. Not good! Fructose is far worse than granulated cane sugar. The United States Department of Agriculture links it directly to obesity and diabetes. And God knows we are certainly a nation of fat people and diabetics. High fructose floods the bowel with undigested carbohydrates and is responsible for 30 to 60% of irritable bowel syndromes. It elevates our LDL or low density lipoproteins commonly referred to as the bad cholesterol. At least with sugar you get a feeling of fullness – not so with fructose. With fructose as we've noted you crave more refined carbohydrates. The remaining three on your list: propylene glycol sodium lauryl sulfate and terpenes have also been covered earlier.

Outside the home there are three major sources of toxins to which we are exposed: prescription drugs, non-prescription drugs (over the counter medications) and the food industry. Make no mistake ALL prescription drugs are toxic and ninety percent of them are not fully metabolized and end up in our water supplies. Currently there are no effective filtering systems to remove them either. According to the American Medical Association prescription drugs are the fourth leading cause of death in America. Think of it. Simply by taking prescription drugs you are increasing your chances of dying by twenty five percent! Certainly not the best odds, I would say. They are also the fourth most common reason for going to a hospital. In my opinion you would do well to discontinue taking any prescription or nonprescription drug. There are alternatives. If you wish to stop taking them you should do so with the knowledge and support of your primary physician. If he/she is not willing to cooperate with your wishes…find another doctor who will be. Over the counter medications aren't much better than prescription drugs from a toxicity standpoint either. Take phenylpropanolamine for example, it was included in many products such as Acutrim, Alka Seltzer, Comtrex, Dexatrim and several kinds of Triaminic before it was finally taken off the market because it was found to produce bleeding in the brain. Such leakage, of course, could lead to serious strokes. NSAIDS or non-steroidal anti-inflammatory drugs that can be purchased over the counter include such things as ibuprofen and aspirins cause 20,000 deaths each year in the United States which is the fifteenth most common cause of death. If they don't kill you, numerous kidney problems could develop. At least 500,000 people a year develop some degree of kidney dysfunction from their continued use.

If our bodies needed these drugs it would make them. Our bodies make antibacterial and antiviral substances.

It possesses a remarkable immune system to fight off disease and makes powerful pain killers too. We don't need toxic chemicals to maintain homeostasis. Homeostasis refers to a balanced state within the body. Most commercial drugs both prescription and non- prescription are synthetic chemicals that try to emulate the beneficial effects of naturally occurring remedies found in nature. MAN was intended to consume live organic foods and not chemicals. Plants do that. For more information regarding toxins and their affect upon humans I recommend the following books:

1. Natural Cures, They Don't Want You To Know About, by Kevin Trudeau
2. Our Toxic World by Doris Rapp, M.D.

It might surprise the daylights out of you to learn that the food industry is a major source of toxins. It starts with farmers who use billions of pounds of pesticides, insecticides, herbicides and fertilizers every year when growing our foodstuffs. There are sixty four common pesticides and of those sixteen cause cancer, twenty four cause brain damage and forty four produce hormonal changes in humans. They are not easy to get rid of either. The United States Department of Agriculture has listed the thirteen most contaminated fruits and vegetables – and this was AFTER WASHING them: (Appendix 'I')

Celery, apples, bell peppers, cherries, grapes (imported), nectarines, Peaches, pears, potatoes, red raspberries, spinach and strawberries.

These insecticides etc. have been found as remote as the North Pole. They dug down a foot deep and still found pesticides like DDT, dioxin and PCB's. While DDT has been outlawed for use in the United States we remain the world's largest producer of it so we are still being exposed as it returns to us on imported fruits and vegetables. Several states dispose of their nuclear waste by mixing it with fertilizers. How thoughtful! An informant at Sloan Kettering Cancer Institute disclosed to the author Kevin Trudeau that every single cancerous tumor analyzed at their center was loaded with insecticides. And the poor farmers themselves are suffering from deep depression, have offspring with birth defects and are dying young of cancer. No one seems to be coming forward to stop this genocide so we must act individually by consuming organically grown foods. The very least we should do is thoroughly wash our fruits and vegetables. June and I soak our produce in a solution of Agricept for about fifteen minutes and then thoroughly rinse them. Agricept is an antivirus, antibacterial, antifungus antiseptic produced from 100% citrus extracts and can be obtained from B&D Marketing-DW, 1490 S. Orange #120 in El Cajon, California 92020.

Dairy cows that are fed hormones produce more milk for sure, but in doing so suffer from swollen udders, ulcers, miscarriages, deformed calves and die quite young – an average of four years earlier than what is considered to be normal. The milk they produce contains blood, pus, tranquilizers, antibiotics and a substance known as insulin growth factor. This innocuous sounding ingredient increases or risk of prostate cancer by four times and breast cancer by seven times. This is the same milk we drink, is used for our school lunch programs and is in our cheeses, yogurts and ice creams. You might think tha all these negatives are erased by Pasteurization. Not really because the toxins are heat resistant and remain. Pasteurization was originally developed to sterilize beer – not milk. It kills bacteria alright but in the process it also destroys enzymes that are necessary for its digestion. This whole scary scenario is also played out with chickens and turkeys and as far as fish farms are concerned the very nicest thing I can say about them is that they are polluted cesspools.

Now let's take a look at the food processor. They are certainly not lily white. Far from it. They put ingredients in our food that makes us hungry so that we buy more groceries. A prime example of such an ingredient would be high fructose corn syrup that we talked about earlier. They also add substances that make us fat. And you know that's working. Just look around you – fat people everywhere! It isn't all due to a lack of exercise. Toxic chemicals such as PCB's used in the processing of food cause hormonal changes in our youngsters – feminization of boys and masculinization of girls. I have often wondered if this might be partly responsible for the apparent increase we are seeing in homosexuality. Over five thousand ingredients are permitted by the FDA to be included in our food products without any mention of them on the labels! How many of those, do you suppose, are toxic?

Seventy five percent of our food is radiated – and has been for ten years or better! I don't know about you, but that concerns the hell out of me. Radiation is dangerous…ask any radiologist. Our bodies do not dissipate radiation any more than they do toxins. Radiation and toxins continue to accumulate throughout our lives. Northwest Nevada to this day continues to have the highest incidence of thyroid cancer as a residual of the atomic tests conducted there several years back. Radiation destroys enzymes, alters the genetic makeup of foods, strips vital nutrients from foods and causes cancer. And, are you ready for this? It goes for your microwave oven too because it cooks by radiation. The microwave oven was invented by the Nazis but researched extensively by the Russians who found them to be extremely dangerous. They alter the molecular structure of foods destroying their quality and forming cancer. You can prove this to yourself. Buy some seeds and plant them in two similar pots. Water one pot with ordinary tap water and the other with water which you have previously 'nuked' in the microwave oven. You will learn that the seeds watered with tap water will germinate but those watered with the 'nuked' water will not. And not so incidentally, cooking food in a microwave oven dramatically raises the level of cholesterol.

And finally there's the grocer who sprays shipping cartons with fungicides and our fruit and vegetables with wax! Is it any wonder why all forms of cancer are on the increase and that we are not winning the war against a single one of them? The simple solution, of course, is to but only organically grown foods. But they, too, should be thoroughly washed.

Now let's have a quick review of the basic food groups: proteins, fats and carbohydrates. You will remember from your school days, I'm sure, that dairy products, meats and vegetables are excellent sources of protein. It comes from the Latin word protos which means first. And protein is first in that it has so many uses in the body. We are all familiar with the fact that protein is necessary for growth and repair of tissue, but it is also useful to make hormones, enzymes and antibodies. All protein is comprised of smaller units called amino acids. When we eat meat or dairy products we break down that protein into amino acids that we then utilize to make our own protein. While on the subject of protein, I'd like to introduce some concerns held by many nutritionists and researchers about pork and pork products. These concerns are apart from any religious considerations. All pork contains retroviruses that cause aids and leukemia. These viruses a very heat resistant and remain for years. Also the lungs of pigs harbor ALL flu viruses – porcine, bird and human. For these reasons you may wish to severely cut back on your consumption of pork.

We obtain fats from essentially the same sources as protein plus of course cooking oils. Fat is an important food group in that it supplies three times more energy than either protein or carbohydrate. Fats are necessary for the absorption of some of the vitamins, it converts carotene into vitamin A and makes hormone like substances called prostaglandins which regulate cellular functions. A shortage of them can result in heart disease, arthritis and/or hormonal deficiencies. They were first isolated from the prostate gland – hence its name – but later it was established that they serve a very important part of every cell function. Omega 3 oils are excellent for making prostaglandins. A saturated fat simply means that it has combined with all the molecules that it can and is differentiated from one that can still combine with other molecules called unsaturated. All animal fat is saturated while most vegetable fat is unsaturated. Humans are better able to digest unsaturated fats than saturated ones simply because unsaturated fats melt at 55 degrees Fahrenheit whereas saturated one melt at 112 degrees. We are also better able to digest cis fats than trans fats. A cis fat is one where all the molecules lie on the same side of a given plane whereas trans fats have molecules on both sides of a plane. Hydrogenated fats are really nothing more than saturated fats since all the molecules have been combined with others by flooding with hydrogen.

There are two basic types of carbohydrates: simple and complex. Simple carbohydrates are also referred to as refined carbohydrates because they are made from refined sugars and flours. Refined carbohydrates are readily absorbed into the blood stream as glucose and tend to make the body acid. The body does not like acid. It tolerates it only within the stomach as it is needed for the digestion of protein and for the absorption of calcium. Otherwise it attempts to neutralize it with alkaline and excrete it. For example, we neutralize carbonic acid and expel it as carbon dioxide when we exhale. Stronger acids are neutralized by a built in mechanism known as the alkaline reserve. This alkaline reserve is established and maintained by eating lots of fruits and vegetables – the rawer the better. The alkaline ash foods and acid ash foods handout that you have is intended to serve as guide for you in planning your meals. Alkaline ash foods should comprise at least seventy five percent of your daily intake. Refined carbohydrates unfortunately comprise everything that tastes so good….cakes, cookies, pies, candy, sugary snacks etc. …but they are all bad for us. They makes us fat, cause diabetes, raise our cholesterol and generally interfere with sound healthful nutrition. They should be avoided at all costs!"

At the conclusion of the seminar several people voiced their appreciation for the new knowledge gained during the session and expressed a desire for future ones. As if on cue, Mrs. Diedrick introduced herself as a member of the school board and practically guaranteed Tom free use of the school auditorium for any future seminar. And finally a gentlemen standing off to the side taking this all in stepped forward and introduced himself as Dick Mills owner of the Deerfield News. He iced the whole idea by offering to run free ads in the newspaper announcing the seminars inasmuch as they would provide a service to the entire community.

Overwhelmed by the outpouring of interest Tom was put into somewhat of an uncompromising position and agreed to conduct at least two more seminars.

"Barbara," he said....

"Yeah, I know. I'll take care of the details."

"Thanks," he said with obvious abasement.

Exercising her usual superior ability and insight Barbara handled all the seminar arrangements with equal ease. They were indeed scheduled in the school auditorium and Mr. Mills was good to his word and ran announcements in the newspaper. The auditorium was sloped from back to front to facilitate a view of the speaker from any seat in the hall. The chairs were cushioned and armed and slid forward and backward to make more room for persons entering or leaving the row. Tom requested the lecturn and microphone be located off stage but centered. The first seminar in the new location dealt with cholesterol and heart disease that was discussed with Bob Holt during one of his office visits and the second dealt with cancer as discussed with Mrs. Mead during one of her visits. Both were very well attended by an estimated seventy five to eighty at the first one and a little over one hundred at the second. The word was getting around.

Tom had always welcomed new innovated methods to improve his service to patients. He was never satisfied with what might be called straight chiropractic and consequently added such modalities as ultrasound, diathermy and electrical stimulation as ancillary treatments to basic spine adjusting. He also became certified in acupuncture further widening his scope of practice and then added the Alpha Stim providing the newly developed microamperage electrical stimulation which has proven to be so highly effective not only in pain management but as a substitute for acupuncture needles. He also became intensely interested in harmful chemicals that we ingest, inject, inhale and absorb on a daily basis. This deep concern was the driving force that sent him on a continual search for more informative facts on the subject. He turned naturally to those who have been practicing alternative and conservative health care medicine for years. He read articles and books and subscribed to monthly newsletters from such notables as Kevin Trudeau, Doris Rapp,M.D., Jonathan Wright, M.D., David Williams, D.C., Julian Whitaker, M.D., and William Campbell Douglass, M.D.. He also joined the Health Sciences Institute that also publishes a monthly newsletter and e-mails important developments on a daily basis. The information that he has gleaned is so noteworthy that it compelled him the 'spread the word' by offering free seminars on a variety of chronic degenerative diseases plaguing mankind. These include arthritis, cancer, heart disease, Alzheimer's disease, osteoporosis and others.

But Tom was not one to throw caution to the wind and when a friend and colleague suggested he attend a seminar on the BEST adjustment he was skeptical and suspicious. Suspicious that it was just another 'low force technique' which he had not embraced in his practiced. He was familiar with Applied Kinesiology, Toffness and Activator procedures but he hadn't incorporated them into his practice either. He decided to attend the seminar yielding to persistent urging by his colleague which included an offer to foot the bill if he felt the material presented was not helpful.

The BEST adjustment was developed and perfected by Dr. Ted Morter. Like so many in the past it was spawned by personal trauma. Dr. Ted was unexpectedly sent soaring by a huge wave while water skiing resulting in a severe neck pain. Where better to have that occur than at a chiropractic convention! Everyone he knew there tried get him some relief by using their 'special techniques' but the many adjustments only seemed to make the pain worse. Even acupuncture was no help. At home Ted went to his own chiropractor and told him to treat him anyway he chose only not to touch his neck. During an adjustment of his sacrum Ted experienced almost instantaneous relief from his neck pain. On the very next day that he was in his office he embarked upon a campaign to find out why his neck pain was helped and yet wasn't touched in the process. The development of the BEST procedure has undergone many refinements and modifications to attain the respectable level of sophistication that it enjoys today.

BEST is an acronym for bio energetic synchronization technique. Magnetic polarity, but not magnets, plays a major role. Briefly the long finger of the right hand emits north energy while the long finger of the left hand emits south energy. Easily remembered as south paw – south energy. That portion of a patients body nearest the earth becomes south so that one lying on his/her stomach (prone) makes it south; conversely a person lying supine or on the back makes it south and the stomach becomes north. Especially tender points are located on the patient through palpation and are treated by placing north and south energy fingers on them and maintaining contact until pulses are detected under each finger. Once pulses are felt the position is held until both pulses are beating at the same rate and intensity. At that point they are synchronized. If other areas of tenderness are palpated and found to be tender they are treated in a similar fashion.

The clearest way to describe the technique simply would be to outline Dr. Morter's demonstration of it as presented in his seminars. Once a doctor is selected from the audience and found to have a cervical subluxation he or she becomes the patient for demonstration purposes. Let's assume for simplicity that one of the bones in the neck has moved very slightly to the left or subluxated left. It is noted that his left leg becomes longer than the right and his left arm weaker than his right one. Arm strength is evaluated by asking a patient to raise an arm straight up into the air while lying on the back or supine. The examiner then tests each arm judging the patient's ability to resist an attempt to pull it downward. It is a very sensitive and reliable test. Next the neck is adjusted by hand using a common technique. The patient is again examined and it is found that both legs are of equal length and both arms equally strong. So far, so good. Then Dr. Morter asks the patient to sit up and lie right back down again. Reexamination shows the legs to once again be unequal in length with the left longer than the right and the left arm has once again become weaker than the right. What happened? Simply that the adjustment did not hold. The brain failed to accept the altered position of the cervical bone. This fact that many adjustments don't hold their positions after adjustment is responsible for one of the most common complaints patients direct toward chiropractors accusing them of repeatedly scheduling appointments that appear to many patients to be unnecessary.

Since the last adjustment failed to hold its position it was predictable that the same disparity between legs and arms prevailed. That is the left leg was long again and the left arm was weak. Dr. Ted then asked the patient to turn over onto his stomach and he began palpating for an acute tender area in the vicinity of the sacrum – not the neck area. It didn't take long before the patient indicated some pain. Ted placed his right long finger on the very spot that induced pain. He then repeated the search process with his left hand underneath the abdomen around the area of the xiphoid process which is a small piece of cartilage projecting downward from the breast bone. Again a tender spot was located and Ted kept his left long finger over it and waited for the two pulses to synchronize after which he searched for other tender areas with which to synchronize. None were found. As a final move he placed his left long finger at the bottom of the coronal suture, which essentially runs across the cranium from ear to ear, and his left index finger above while his right long finger (north energy) remained on the tender spot of the sacrum and waited for those three pulses to synchronize. (If the left long finger is south energy then the left index finger must be north energy otherwise the fingers would be repelled.) When the patient turned over on his back again, Ted once again evaluated leg length and arm strength. As expected both legs were of equal length and both arms equally strong. He then asked the patient to sit up and lie back down again as before and reexamined. No change was noted. Both legs were even and both arms strong. Fifteen or twenty minutes later into the seminar he called the patient up to the front again and reexamined him. No change. The adjustment was still holding and amazingly he never touched the patients neck!

It should be noted that the pulses felt are not vascular in nature but rather are cellular. That is when the female egg, which is beating at a distinct rate, meets and unites with the male sperm, which also has its own pulse rate, a new and separate pulse is developed which is subsequently passed on to every cell in your body – all seventy to seventy five trillion of them. "This man has got something," Tom thought and that conviction carried through three additional seminars that Tom needed no prodding to attend.He then began to include BEST in his armamentarium. His first opportunity to employ BEST came from a gentlemen with a frozen shoulder. He had been to an orthopedic surgeon and even tried acupuncture to no avail. Tom treated him basically as described above finishing up with a double crown over the coronal suture and another contact on an acutely tender spot of the shoulder as pointed out by the patient. Tom never saw him again but decided to call him several months later as a follow up.

"After you treated me the pain left and I immediately regained full use of my shoulder. I haven't been back to see you because I haven't needed you." Wow, Tom said to himself. That's amazing. What a nice way to lose a patient..

Another case was even more amazing. Nancy H… was being treated for back pain incurred as a result of an automobile accident. She had been driving a van and was hit in the middle of an intersection on the passenger side. Tom was treating her with acupuncture and almost as an after thought decided to try a BEST adjustment after acupuncture. During the next office visit Nancy expressed a desire to be treated exclusively by BEST as she felt she had gotten more relief from it than acupuncture. And she did respond very nicely and the back pain disappeared. Tom was all set to release her from treatment when he inadvertently asked if she had pain anywhere else.

"No," she said, "just in the leg."

"What leg?" Tom asked.

"I told you about my accident." Tom acknowledged that but wasn't aware that she had leg pain along with back pain. She explained that she was thrown against the door handle or window crank when she was hit from the side. The accident occurred in January or February and we were treating her in August. Tom asked her to point to the pain and he covered it with north energy and simultaneously took a double crown contact over the coronal suture. He explained that he was going to release her but that she had better return again later in the week so he could evaluate the pain in her leg. She did return and when Tom went into her treatment room she said she had something to show him. With that she lifted her skirt to expose a bruise on her left leg that measured fully four inches wide and eight inches long. Even Tom threw his head backward in dismay. Never before nor since had he ever seen a bruise that large. Then she amazed him even more by saying that the pain was gone!! Miraculous that's what it was. Apparently Tom's treatment sent new sensory information to her brain which decided that the pain in her leg was no longer necessary but the same bruise that she suffered after the accident reappeared. Gradually the bruise subsided and Nancy was fine.

Tom was already standing behind the lectern arranging his notes as the school auditorium was filling up rapidly. When things quieted down a bit he turned the microphone on and surveyed the audience until there was complete silence.

"Good evening, ladies and gentlemen. Thank you for coming. Tonight we will be covering the bony subjects of arthritis and osteoporosis. As always I sincerely hope that you will be able to derive some benefit from the information presented."

"First let's take a look at arthritis. It may be belaboring the obvious a bit but in order to have arthritis a joint must be involved. You would be surprised at the number of patients that would point to a painful spot between the shoulder and elbow or between the hip and knee and ask me if I thought it could be arthritis. Often a bruised bone or muscle strain is mistaken for arthritis. I might interject here the difference between a strain and a sprain. A strain involves a tendon which attaches a muscle to a bone. A sprain involves a ligament which attaches a bone to another bone. No muscle is involved here. The reason a sprain takes so long to heal is that ligaments as a whole have a poor blood supply so that healing nutrients are slow in coming to an injured area. A muscle has a very generous blood supply and consequently a strain heals much faster.

It might be helpful for a better understanding of just what arthritis is to cover a little anatomy. A joint consists of two bones in close proximity to one another but not normally touching. The end of each bone is covered with a thin layer of cartilage which is bathed in a fluid called synovial fluid. The entire joint is encased by a fibrous capsule. Synovial fluid is a very important part of a joint not only cushioning it but in supplying vital nutrients for it. You see, cartilage does not have any blood supply whatsoever and must receive its nutrients from surrounding tissues which in this case is synovial fluid.

So what does arthritis do to all this anatomy, anyway? There is a loss of synovial fluid through leakage or failure to replenish itself followed by erosion and eventual destruction of the cartilage covering the ends of the bones. The area is loaded with pain receptors known as nocioreceptors and pain is the normal result. This gradual erosion of a joint helps to explain how and why arthritis is progressive. The body tries its best to heal the area and prevent further damage but sooner or later yields to overwhelming destruction.

Radioactive studies have shown that human bone should last for 120 years. So why would God have our gall bladders fail at age 45 and our bones go to hell around age 70? He didn't, of course. MAN in his infinite wisdom has taken care of that. You and I have talked before about the enormous amount of toxins we ingest, inject, inhale and absorb on a daily basis. These are ALL man made. They are not at all natural. So certainly our continuous marriage with these toxins has been most instrumental in causing many of the chronic degenerative diseases that are plaguing mankind today not the least of which is arthritis. The causes of arthritis are many and varied. There are several types of bacteria that seem to attack joints and lend their names to the type of arthritis. For example, there is gonococcal arthritis, tubercular arthritis named from the gonococcus and tuberculin bacillae respectively. Streptococcus can produce rheumatic fever and affect joints. There are also special types of arthritis named after individuals who first described them such as Sjorgren's and Reiter's triads. By far the most common types, however, are osteoarthritis and rheumatoid arthritis which we'll talk about in a little more detail shortly. Dr. David Williams places a lot of emphasis upon deficiencies as a primary cause. He mentions such deficiencies as vitamins and minerals and vital nutrients. He also claims that nitrates in fried foods especially in fast food restaurants is a frequent cause and probably has contributed to the dramatic increase in the disease. Dr. Jonathan Wright feels that aging and overuse are not nearly the influential cause as some authors suggest but that the toxic chemicals used to both grow our foods and process them probably represents the major cause of all types of arthritis. Some people have food allergies because of the addition of these toxic chemicals which disappear when eating organic foods. Food allergies as a cause of arthritis ranks pretty highly.

Osteoarthritis is far and away the most common type of arthritis we see here in America. Unlike rheumatoid arthritis it affects one side of the body. That's not to say that one couldn't have arthritis of the right thumb for example and also of the left hip – but not the left thumb. If you have rheumatoid arthritis of an elbow it affects both elbows at the same time. Osteoarthritis is considered to be non-inflammatory but sometimes a joint can be so irritated that a little inflammation does result. It, however, is not a flaming hot inflammation that can be felt to the touch as with rheumatoid. When the hand is affected there is no deformation but characteristic nodules can appear at the furthest or distal knuckle(s) of the fingers called Heberden's nodules. Rheumatoid arthritis is considered to be an autoimmune disease which simply means that for some reason the body's immune system begins to attack its normal tissues. As we have noted it affects both sides of the body at the same time, is quite inflammatory, can cause deforming and create nodules that are not limited to the distal knuckles but can appear almost anywhere. You may recall noticing such deformity in the hands of Lionel Barrymore and John Carradine in some of the movies in which they appeared.

The mainstream medical approach to treating arthritis is pretty much the same as anything else – drugs and surgery. The drugs consist mainly of COX2 inhibitors and NSAIDs. COX2 is a destructive enzyme producing inflammation and inhibiting drugs are used to counteract it. You may recall our previous discussions regarding NSAIDs that can create havoc with both the liver and kidneys and even cause death due to excessive use of them. Recall, too, that they include a class of drugs known as ibuprofens such as Motrin and Advil. Before these drugs can become active and effective they must form a complex with copper. If you are in the habit of using these drugs on a regular basis it might pay you to add some copper to your diet lest it be depleted by forming these complexes with ibuprofen drugs.

Although osteoarthritis and rheumatoid arthritis share some similarities as far as treatment with alternative and conservative approaches there are some distinct differences and therefore will be discussed separately. First osteoarthritis. Jonathan Wright, M.D. reminds us that eliminating certain vegetables known as 'nightshade vegetables' can frequently bring welcome relief to arthritis sufferers. These plants are generally from warm climates and have a round stem, rank smell and a watery sap and include the tobaccos, red peppers, tomatoes, potatoes, petunias and egg plants. Some people are quite sensitive to them, can not metabolize them and develop arthritis as a result. At the present time there is no test available to determine one's susceptibility to these vegetables other than eliminating them to see if the osteoarthritis is relieved. This can take three or four months of abstinence. Similarly some cases of osteoarthritis can be aggravated by certain food allergies and it might pay one to undergo a food allergy screening. Probably the most common ingredient for treating osteoarthritis has been glucosamine which is a naturally occurring stimulant for cartilage growth. Some manufacturers have combined it with chondroitin and others have even added a third ingredient called methylsulfonylmethane or simply MSM. Chondroitin has come under fire recently as possibly causing cancer. So if you are currently taking it you might want to consider discontinuing it until the matter becomes sorted out. Some manufacturers have also added medicinal herbs to their products and I have listed three of them if you'd care to take note:

TheraFlex
1.800.270.4881
adds 14 herbs

ArthriPhase
Tango Advanced Nutrition
1.866.778.2646
adds 12 herbs

OlyJoint
Bio Nutrigenics

1.888.330.4372
glucosamine, chondroitin and MSM
adds 2 herbs

Niacinamide, not plain niacin, works very well for pain and inflammation of joints affected with arthritis. It doesn't seem to aid in the growth of cartilage or its repair so it is recommended that glucosamine be taken along with it. Dr. Wright recommends 1000 mg. three times a day along with 500 mg. of glucosamine. Other remedies that you may wish to discuss with your conservative healthcare professional are as follow:

For pain: Boswellia
           Ashwaganda
           Willow bark
For inflammation: Bromelain
                  Curcumin
                  Gamma linolenic acid
                  Quercetin

A word about the use of plain niacin is warranted. Niacin has worked very well indeed against pain and inflammation. The problem involves the tolerance, or I should say the intolerance, that most people have to it. It produces a flush throughout which is often followed by terrible itching. It can take a person quite a long time to overcome these 'side effects' and many give up before the body adapts. Anyway, 250 mg. of niacin taken every two hours for eight doses has been quite helpful in even severe cases of arthritis. For extreme cases the dosage can be increased to every one and a half hours for ten doses. Time release capsules to avoid flushing and itching are not recommended because they have a tendency to create serious liver problems.

Allergies seem to play an even larger role in cases of rheumatoid arthritis than they do with ostoarthritis. Milk and dairy products are major culprits and should be ruled out first during any allergy evaluation. Some rheumatoid sufferers have experienced great relief simply by eliminating dairy products. Many reliable studies have shown that rheumatoid arthritic patients have low levels of hydrochloric acid which you will remember is necessary for protein digestion and the absorption of calcium. Fish oils are more important in the treatment of rheumatoid arthritis than they are for osteoarthritis. These should always be supplemented with vitamin E. Some healthcare professionals might also medicate with ginger, zinc, copper and selenium all of which have been found to be helpful.

Let's stop here for a few minutes and stretch our legs before talking about osteoporosis."

Now, let's go on to osteoporosis. Osteoporosis medically is a loss of bone density which makes the bone quite brittle and subject to more frequent fracturing. Approximately ten million people are affected and of those eight million are women who are most affected after menopause. It may be linked to a relative increase in estrogen when progesterone levels decrease during menopause. Or perhaps it's due to a decline of DHEA during menopause. DHEA or dehydroepiandrosterone is a hormone produced by the ovaries as well as the adrenal glands that has been shown to have a bone building effect. It is believed that DHEA plays a more important role in the prevention of osteoporosis than does estrogen. But be that as it may it doesn't correlate well with the fact that we are seeing osteoporosis in thirty year old men and women.

When you think of bone the only mineral that comes to mind, of course, is calcium. It should be noted that in order for calcium to be absorbed by the body both hydrochloric acid and vitamin D are required. There alone we have some possible factors leading to osteoporosis. Magnesium and cholesterol are necessary to produce vitamin D. Processing foods strips them of magnesium and statin drugs reduce cholesterol. Processing foods also strips vitamin D from them and finally the tons of antacids consumed in this country reduces the amount of hydrochloric acid. All in all these represent areas that could interfere with the absorption of calcium. There are other factors that reduce calcium absorption such as too much caffeine and high salt diets which are contributed to greatly by processed foods.

Many of us have been led to believe that milk is a good source of calcium. There are at least three indisputable facts that belie this propaganda from the Milk Institute.

1. Pasteurization, which was developed to sterilize beer, destroys harmful bacteria to be sure but it also destroys enzymes necessary to digest milk.
2. The calcium/phosphorous ratio in humans is 2.5 to 1; that is to say we require two and a half times more calcium than phosphorous. In cows the ratio is 1 to 1. So when we drink cows milk we actually have a greater need for calcium than before we drank it in order to satisfy our ratio.
3. As soon as infants begin cutting their teeth, they lose an enzyme called rennin which is necessary for its assimilation. This rennin is not to be confused with the renin produced in the kidneys and note that it is spelled with two n's. Cow's milk is for baby cows and not humans!

Now, let's turn to animal protein as distinguished from vegetable protein. In a previous seminar we mentioned that a high protein diet is desirable followed by fats and finally carbohydrates and that most of the protein should be derived from vegetables and not meat. Too much animal protein is not good for us because as we digest it and use certain amino acids to make our own protein three rather strong acids are produced: nitric, phosphoric and sulfuric. You may recall from our previous seminars that the body does not like acid. The only place it wants acid is in the stomach to aid in the digestion of protein and the absorption of calcium that we discussed earlier this evening. The body wants to be alkaline. Blood is alkaline. Digestive enzymes are alkaline and so are lymph and bile. We should be happy that the body wants to be in an alkaline state because viruses and cancer cells cannot exist in an alkaline environment. What this has to do with bone and osteoporosis will become clear in a moment. But first let's address just how the body gets rid of unwanted acid. One way is to breathe. When we exhale carbon dioxide we are ridding the body of carbonic acid. You probably see people jogging everyday. They may be sweating bullets and have pain written all over their faces but by golly they're going to run come rain or snow. Why on earth? Because when they finish they feel like a million dollars simply because they have rid themselves of a lot of acid. Personally, I could sit and watch them all day long. But breathing does not get rid of stronger acids such as those developed when protein is digested. They have to be neutralized by equal amounts of alkaline to form neutral salts that can be easily eliminated by the kidneys. And I am not referring to Alka Seltzer either. No, we have a built in mechanism called the alkaline reserve which is established and maintained by eating plenty of fruits and vegetables – the rawer the better. But if the presence of acids becomes overwhelming the alkaline reserve can't keep up and soon will be depleted. When that occurs the body will go to the bone and leech out calcium. Too much of that and bingo we have osteoporosis. It's been shown if we consume more than six ounces of animal protein or meat per day the body will leech calcium from bones. Which bones? The smaller ones first such as those in the hands, feet and spine. This limitation of six ounces of meat per day holds true whether or not you eat extra portions of fruits and vegetables.

You might consider adding some strontium to your diet. It has been shown to increase bone density. Vitamin K2 also bonds calcium to bone and has the unique property of not depositing it in arteries. Green vegetables such as spinach, broccoli and asparagus are good sources of vitamin K2. Finally you would do well to curtail your consumption of cola drinks – diet or otherwise. They are very high in phosphorus which interferes with calcium metabolism.

We have covered quite a lot of material this evening and I'll be glad to answer any questions that you might have." With that invitation hands flew up all over the auditorium and Tom spent the next half hour or so answering their questions and listening to their comments.

The school auditorium which holds about 350 people was nearly half full again of patients and guests anxiously waiting for another inspiring seminar conducted by Dr. Clayton. Tom rose from a chair in front of the stage, walked to the lectern where he switched on the microphone and then waited for the audience to quiet down. He then spoke: "Larry went into a neighborhood saloon about 9:58 P.M. for a nightcap. The placed was packed and he claimed the last stool at the bar which happened to be next to a gorgeous blonde. Just about that time the ten o'clock news came on the television set above the bar. It was featuring a man standing on top of a tall building threatening to commit suicide. Larry turned to the blonde sitting next to him and said 'I'll bet he jumps.'

'I've got ten bucks that says he doesn't.' she replied. No sooner had she said that and the guy jumped off the building to his death. 'Well I'll be damned,' she said as she pushed her ten dollars toward Larry.

'I can't take your money,' he replied. 'I knew that he jumped because I saw the five o'clock news.' A few laughs came from the audience.

'Well, I did too,' she said, 'but I didn't think he'd do it again.' The audience then broke out into hilarious laughter."

"Thank you for coming," Tom continued. "Tonight we'll be discussing the evils of sugar including diabetes. It will also be our last seminar of the series." Almost immediately there was a nearly unanimous groan of disappointment throughout the hall. "Well maybe we'll repeat them next year provided we have enough fresh material to keep it interesting." The comment was met a resounding applause of approval.

"Maybe we had better get started before I think of another joke." A few giggles could be heard coming from the audience as Tom continued. " Excess consumption of sugar has been, in my opinion, accurately described as slow suicide. Not like jumping off a roof but just as lethal. Sugar has no nutritional value, contains no vitamins or minerals, has no useful calories and is no good for us. It makes us fat and can cause diabetes. It also combines with body proteins in the absence of anti-oxidants in a process known as glycation that causes all kinds of problems like heart attacks, strokes, kidney failure, cataracts, destruction of blood vessels and nerves and produces amyloid plaques in Alzheimer's disease. Bad stuff. This glycation process of sugar and body proteins produces 'advanced glycation end products' known best by its acronym AGE's.

Fructose, high fructose, corn syrup or whatever you choose to call it is no better than sugar and in some respects even worse. HFCS was introduced into our food supply about the same time as the infamous hydrogenated oils. When the widespread use began in the 1970's, the obesity rate was stable but from that point on it began to rise steadily and by 2000 it had doubled. It continues to grow to this day. Dr. Williams states that we experience some of the highest rates of disease and lowest life expectancy rates of any industrialized nation on Earth. At least when you consume sugar you experience a full feeling and it helps to suppress your hunger. Fructose does neither one of these and in fact actually increases your desire for more of it. The United States Department of Agriculture has established a strong link between fructose and obesity as well as diabetes. Fructose has been shown to increase LDL or low density lipoproteins. It floods the bowel with undigested carbohydrates causing 'irritable bowel syndromes'. Authorities differ as to the degree of incidence with some indicating only 30% being attributed to fructose while others claim as high as 60%. The food industry is notorious in its use as a sweetener in thousands upon thousands of food products. Check your labels carefully. It is present even in dry cereals – along with sugar, of course. Maybe

Kevin Trudeau is right in suggesting we don't purchase anything in a jar, box or bag that is produced by a major food company that is publicly traded. They are far more concerned with their stockholders than they are with your health.

From where does all this sugar come? We're going to take a look at 'hidden sugars' later but for now let's concentrate upon those sugars for which we have some control. I refer, of course, to simple sugars found in refined carbohydrates. Sugars such as sucrose, glucose, maltose and lactose are very quickly digested and absorbed into the blood. Sugar in the blood is called glycemia – glyc coming from Greek meaning 'sweet'and emia always refers to blood. You will then recognize the familiar terms of hyperglycemia and hypoglycemia referring to excessive and insufficient sugar in the blood respectively. A normal range for blood sugar is 80 to 100 mg./dl. A deciliter is approximately three and a third ounces. These refined carbohydrates are found in foods such as pies, cakes, cookies, snacks, donuts etc. ad infinitum. All of these are delicious and often present a serious challenge to avoid eating too much of them. But control them we must in order to maintain a proper blood sugar balance and avoid gaining weight and/or running the risk of contracting diabetes. And don't forget the dangers of 'glycation end products'. We don't want to be guilty of slighting complex carbohydrates. These include such things as potatoes, beans, lentils and grains. Complex carbohydrates are digested and absorbed more slowly than simple ones but they do contribute glucose to the blood.

An oft repeated adage has insulin 'burning' sugar to produce energy. Don't fall for that one. Insulin, a hormone produced by the pancreas gland, plays an important role in the metabolism of all our food groups – proteins, fats and carbohydrates. It stores sugar in the form of glycogen in the liver and all muscles and turns any excess sugar into fat. Its major role, though, is to move sugar from the blood stream into cells which in turn convert it into energy. For a little bit of trivia; glucose is the only food utilized by the brain – and no, eating a lot of candy will not make you smarter! It will be helpful to learn at this point that every cell in your body contains receptors for insulin. Think of them as little doorways. Chromium and water soluble cinnamon have been shown to increase the sensitivity of these receptors or little doorways and are used by some doctors in the regulation of blood sugar in diabetic patients as well as those considered to be at risk.

Let's talk about low blood sugar or hypoglycemia for a minute. This condition is rather common today because of the widespread craving for refined carbohydrates which, you will remember, very quickly turn to sugar. On an average we consume 152 pounds of sugar per year. That may not sound like a lot to you but it equates to about 14,500 teaspoons a year or about 40 teaspoons a day. And that's an average remember. Some of us consume more. Anyway it puts a great demand upon the pancreas to secrete insulin which usually rises to the occasion and removes sugar from the blood stream. It's easy to deduce, then, that an ever increasing demand for insulin could result in low blood sugar or hypoglycemia. People with hypoglycemia are sluggish most of the time, tire easily especially after meals, are filled with ennui and may even be a little slow mentally. The cells are crying for some sugar but there's not enough left in the blood to meet the demand. In that situation the pancreas secretes yet another hormone called glucagon (sounds like glucose gone) which metabolizes fat deposits for energy. Wow! A good way to lose weight? Not really, but if you like the idea of decreasing fat deposits to supply energy allow me to introduce CLA or conjugated linoleic acid. A major source of CLA is from open range fed cattle. Since those cattle are not very prevalent in this country, CLA can be purchased from your friendly health food store. One product with which I am familiar is called Tonalin. If you decide to go this route be prepared to give it some time – 3 months or more might pass before you notice some results in weight loss. Don't expect liposuction results. Be patient. Why does it take so long before you notice any results? Mobilizing fat is not the only role it plays. It is also busy helping insulin move glucose into cells, aids in immunity and even helps to retard the growth of cancerous tumors within the prostate gland.

Okay, now let's take a look at diabetes. Dr. Wright tells us that with it's complications it is the third leading cause of death in the United States. The term comes from a 'flowing through' from the Latin dia or through and in this case a flowing through the kidneys. We should differentiate between diabetes insipidus and diabetes mellitus. Diabetes insipidus is a loss of fluid through frequent urination because the kidneys fail to reabsorb water which is a normal function of them. Diabetes mellitus is a loss of fluid as well as sugar in the urine. This is the one with which we are concerned tonight. Some warning signs that might herald diabetes mellitus are skin spots, skin tags, excessive weight, sores that fail to heal and an uncontrollable flexion of a finger called Dupuytren's contracture. A British study indicates that persons taking beta blocker drugs increase the risk of developing diabetes by fifty percent because they shut down the pancreas' production of insulin. If you are currently a diabetic you have a lot of company according to The World Health Organization that estimate there are 171 million others suffering from the disease. Worse they expect that number to double by 2030. So like so many other chronic degenerative diseases diabetes mellitus is on the increase.

From where does the sugar in the urine come? Diabetics are hyperglycemic with blood sugar levels something over 100 mg/dl which is considered to be at the high end of normal. The blood has so much sugar that it cannot contain it without spilling it over into the urine. The sugar that does spill over into the urine was not able to be delivered to cells for basically three reasons:

1. Insufficient insulin
2. Cells are too sick to accept sugar
3. The insulin receptors have become insensitive

Many diabetics are able to control their blood sugar levels by careful dieting while others require insulin either taken orally or by injection. Most diabetics have an excess of insulin in their blood called hyperinsulinemia because the body attempts to produce more to drive glucose into the cells which become desensitized at the receptors. This all has a tendency to elevate the blood pressure, too. I hope you remember our discussion regarding glycation and the formation of glycation end products or AGE's. These glycation end products stiffen blood vessels elevating blood pressure and causing eye problems, heart attacks and strokes. AGE's also destroy nerves as well. So you see uncontrolled blood sugar levels can really cause serious problems.

None of this applies to me, you might think because you don't consume much sugar. Maybe and maybe not. I could have some very disturbing news for you." Tom moved away from behind the lectern to a table containing an overhead projector and turned it on. "We're going to look at some overheads that will drive home the fact that the food industry is loading its products with tons of 'hidden sugars'. (Appendix 'F'). Soda pop including ginger ale contains 5 teaspoons of sugar. Sweet cider is even worse at 6 teaspoons full. A 4 oz. piece of chocolate cake with icing has 10 teaspoons of sugar in it. One ginger snap has 3 teaspoons full. A macaroon and a glazed donut contain 6 teaspoons of sugar in them. Look at hard candy. Four ounces contain 20 teaspoons of sugar and that's equivalent to ten Hershey bars! By comparison canned fruits and juices are not so bad. Ice cream products vary from three to seven teaspoons of sugar. Jams and jellies contain anywhere from four to six teaspoons of sugar – and that's without taking in to account the added fructose. Look at the leading cereals. They're not shown in relation to teaspoons of sugar but a percentage of the entire product. One of my favorites is Nabisco's 100% Bran. Notice that almost 20% of that product is sugar! Another is Quaker's 100% Natural. It contains a little over 17% sugar. So you see, you may be thinking only what sugar you consume at the dinner table and not taking into account the amount added by the food industry who are desperately trying to 'hook' you into buying more and more sweet tasting products. Also remember the ingredients are listed on a package in the order of their volume content. Some list both sugar and fructose in the same product!! It's all about money.

Tom acknowledged a raised hand, "Yes sir, do you have a question or comment?"

"Yes. I realize this is your last seminar of the year but I have a mother who has been diagnosed with Alzheimer's disease and I would certainly appreciate your taking some more time to comment on the subject. If the others here tonight are not in accord, I will be happy to make an appointment at your office for a consultation." Addressing the audience Tom asked if they would like to spend some time now for discussion or wait until next year sometime. A round of approving applause along with a few "let's do it now" voices settled the matter. After a short stretch break Tom called the seminar to order as he approached the podium.

"In order to better understand memory loss and specifically Alzheimer's disease it would be most helpful o have a short course in neuroanatomy so that we can at least understand how nerve impulses are propagated." As he spoke To flipped n an overhead projector, lowered a large screen for viewing and began to draw figure 'A' on a sheet of acetate. (Appendix 'H'). This is what a typical nerve cell or neuron looks like. These appendages stand-out prominently unlike any other cell. This one on the right side is known as the axon. A neuron has only one of those and it transmits impulses AWAY from the cell. All the other appendages are called dendrites because they re-semble a tree and they transmit impulses TO the body or soma of the neuron. These thin strands represent nerve fibers and the button like structures at their ends repre-sent a connection with the neuron called a synapse." To set figure 'A' aside and began drawing figure 'B'. This is an enlargement of a single synapse of a nerve fiber mak-ing connection in this case with the soma or body of the neuron. Bear in mind, however, that synapses are made with dendrites as well. At the end of each nerve fiber there are several small vesicles filled with chemicals that transmit impulses across the synapses and are called neu-rotransmitters. Cell bodies and dendrites are well sup-plied with receptors to receive these chemicals. This is the process by which a nerve impulse is propagated or moved forward from one nerve to another. The most prevalent neurotransmitter is a chemical called acetyl-choline which you might glean from its name is made from cholesterol.

You can appreciate that if anything were to disrupt or block the release of acetylcholine from the nerve ending the movement or propagation of an impulse would be impaired or compromised. If the impulse happens o be memory one then, some memory could be lost. This is essentially what happens in Alzheimer's disease. Many of the toxins that we have discussed that cause chronic degenerative diseases also can cause neurologic disorders. I refer specifically to insecticides, pesticides, prescription and non prescription drugs, and chemicals used in processing our foods. For example anticholinergic drugs which block acetylcholine causing memory loss, dementia and Alzheimer's disease are in very common use in many medications used to treat asthma, over active bladders, gastrointestinal cramps, diarrhea, pain, anxiety, seizures, high blood pressure, heart failure, arthritis and Parkinson's disease. That's quite a list, isn't it? To me, is another example of man's inhumanity toward man.

Let's talk about lithium for a minute. Most of us recognize lithium as a trace mineral that has been used for decades in severe mental conditions. More and more evidence, though, points to its effectiveness in other neurologic conditions – in much smaller doses however. It has been shown to have encouraging results not only in Alzheimer's disease but in cases of amyotrophic lateral sclerosis better known as ALS or Lou Gehrigs disease and Parkinson's disease. Lithium protects neurons by helping them to regenerate axons and increase the number of brain cells.

Alzheimer's disease is but one o some 70 dementias and is projected to affect 20% of the adult population over 65 years of age. It is quite rare in India while on the increase here in America. What is India doing that we are not or vice versa? We'll find out shortly. One of the changes in the brain of an Alzheimer's victim is the deposition of amyloid plaques that affect memory. (Appendix 'I'). One possible explanation for these plaques is that they are actually AGE's an acronym for advanced glycation end products that are formed by a combination of a sugar with a protein. You may recall our previous discussions of this phenomena and the fact that AGE's can be very destructive to both blood vessels and nerves. I have often wondered if AGE's was a factor in President Reagan's bout with Alzheimer's. since he was an avid jelly bean consumer. In Alzheimer's patients memory impulses are destroyed before crossing synapses by another chemical called cholinesterase. Therefore by inhibiting cholinesterase impulses can be prolonged and memory impulses lengthened in duration. This is the concept behind orthodox medicines approach but the drugs have severe side effects such as liver damage, seizures and deep depression. They are also rather short lived losing their effectiveness within a year.

Recognizing that there are no known cures for Azheimer's disease let's take a look at some alternative approaches that don't have any such severe reactions as prescription drugs. A link between Alzheimer's and aluminum is controversial. Some believe a distinct link exists while others discard it entirely. We do know that fluorine enhances the accumulation of aluminum while silicon decreases it. There are currently four alternative treatments with which I am familiar that halt the progression of the disease. These are huperzine which is a Chinese herb and powerful cholinesterase inhibitor; alpha lipoic acid (ALA); galantamine which is a plant extract and acts similarly to ALA in halting progression; and lithium which inhibits the formation of amyloid plaques and neurofibril tangles. Dr. Jonathan Wright has been treating Alzheimer's patients with lithium asparatate or lithium orotate for several years with great success. For years now alternative health care professionals have known that ALA stops the progression of Alzheimer's with 600 mg/day along with 300 mcg/day of biotin. Researchers now believe that ALA may also be beneficial in retarding cataracts as well as the symptoms of Parkinson's disease. Galatamine, which mimics ALA remember, has been widely used in fifteen different countries in Europe and has been approved by our FDA. It is not widely used here, and won't be, because it is natural and can not be patented and sold for billions of dollars by big pharma. Other treatments include curcumin which is the main ingredient of curry, a popular food in India. Curcumin protects the brain from amyloid plaque formation. Now you know why Indians have fewer Alzheimer's patients than we. Though a little expensive acetyl L- carnitine available in health food stores slows the deterioration of neurons. Plain old lecithin has been found to be clinically comparable to the prescription drug Donepezil which runs around $120.00 per month.

I hope your neurons are functioning up to par and you won't forget the things we've talked about tonight!!

It was a beautiful Sunday without a cloud in the sky, temperatures hovering around 75 degrees and low humidity. A perfect day for a graduation. In sharp contrast to Jenny's graduation two years earlier which was nearly ruined by torrential rains. Some gusts of wind had to be at least 50 miles an hour. Saplings struggling to remain rooted nearly formed inverted 'U's. Heavy patio furniture was moved by the strong winds in a wraith- like manner from place to place. Bamboo blinds, although rolled up tightly, were blown from their foundations. The wind was predictably followed by proverbial sheets of rain so hard that they literally distorted some views and obscured others. The deluge tested the caulking seals of skylights and small puddles of water that formed beneath them gave testimony to the forces behind the rain. Today though on a nice sunny and mild day Bill will be receiving his doctorate in chiropractic medicine. Five long and hard years of intense study culminated in a forty five minute ceremony. Bill had been elected class president who's duty it was to deliver an inspiring speech to his classmates at graduation. And inspiring it was. He had researched the many challenges confronting the profession in the past, drew analogies with present ones and challenged his classmates to become active within the profession pointing to their willingness as the greatest challenge of them all. He was interrupted a couple of times during his delivery with applause of approval and later in the ceremony the college president made reference to some of Bill's remarks during his address. As class president Bill was the first to graduate even before the valedictorian. The college president called Bill's name and then announced that his father, Dr. Thomas Clayton, would assist in the hooding process. A hood is a silky type of cloth that loosely wraps around the throat and drapes down the back displaying the school's color which in this case is red and makes a striking contrast with the traditionally black gown. As Bill and his father walked off the stage the Dean of Students handed Bill his diploma, shook his hand while congratulating him as well as his father. Dr. William Clayton. Has a nice ring to it, Bill thought.

Later at home June and Tom had invited a few close friends who had known Bill through his formative years right into college to drop in and celebrate Bill's graduation. June had prepared some triangular finger sandwiches and Tom tended bar. Gifts were deliberately excluded. It was a comfortable and relaxing affair after the excitement and commotion connected with a graduation ceremony. After the company had left all the Claytons busied themselves with the chore of cleaning up the dishes and straightening things up a bit. Tom asked Bill if he had given any thought as to what he was going to do now.

"Well Dad, you've mentioned a couple of times that you'd like to see me come in with you. Is that still an option for you?"

"You betcha. I couldn't be more excited about the idea. I didn't wish to make a large issue of it because I wanted it to be your decision and not what you thought I wanted. We have plenty of room at the office and until you develop a practice that occupies most of your time if you'd like you can shadow me and even assist with treatments."

"Gee," Bill said with a grin, "I'll be learning from the greatest."

" I envy your experience," Tom said returning a grin. With arms around the other's shoulders they headed for the kitchen.

Appendix 'A'

Natural Methods To Reduce Cholesterol

1. Niacin
2. Omega 3 oils
3. Vitamin C (mega doses)
4. Policosonol
5. Tocotrienols (vitamin E complex)
6. Arjuna
7. Nattokinase
8. Discard all microwaves
9. Lecithin
10. Red yeast rice (caution: it contains the same basic molecule found in statin drugs)

Appendix 'B'

Natural Ways To Prevent Heart Disease

1. Antioxidants
2. 400+ I.U.'s of vitamin E
3. Magnesium
4. Reduce sugar consumption
5. Vitamin C (mega doses)
6. Celery (4 to 5 stalks)
7. Blood thinners:
   a. Omega 3 oils
   b. Magnesium
   c. Vitamin E
   d. Garlic
   e. Policosonol
   f. Bromelain
   g. Tocotrienols
   h. L-Arginine
8. Vitamin D
9. Vitamin K2

Appendix 'C'

Examples Of Things To Avoid
for a
Healthier Disease-Free Life

Compiled by
Robert T. Story, D.C.

Acid ash foods
Alcohol (excessive)
Aspartame
Cell phones
Chlorine
Diethylanolamine
Diethylstilbesterol
Farm fish
Fluorine
Fructose
Glycol esters
Hexachlorophene
Hydrogenated oils
Microwave
Non-prescription drugs & medications
Pasteurized milk
Pork
Prescription drugs

Processed food
Propylene glycol
Radiated foods
Refined carbohydrates
Sodium lauryl sulfate
Soy
Sugar
Terpenes
Trans fats

Appendix 'D'

Examples Of Foods That Leave
An Alkaline Residue
(listed in order of their positive effect)

Raw spinach	Cauliflower
Beet greens	Pineapple
Molasses	Avocado
Celery	Raisons
Dried figs	Dried dates
Carrots	Green beans
Dried beans	Limes
Chard leaves	Sour cherries
Watercress	Tangerines
Sauerkraut	Strawberries
Lettuce	White potato
Lima beans	Sweet potato
Rhubarb	Grapefruit
Cabbage	Apricot
Broccoli	Lemon
Beets	Blackberries
Brussels sprouts	Oranges
Cucumbers	Tomatoes
Parsnips	Peaches
Radishes	Raspberries
Drjed peas	Banana
Mushrooms	Onions

Grapes
Pears
Blueberries
Apples
Watermelon
Green peas

Appendix 'E'

Examples Of Foods That
Leave An Acid Residue
(listed in increasing order)

Corn syrup
Olive oil
Corn oil
Sugar
Fresh corn
Honey
Pork chops
Whole wheat bread
Eggs
Bacon
Lamb chops
English walnuts
Wheat bran
White bread
Lamb
Veal chops
Barley
Turkey
Beefsteak
Salmon
White flour
Whole wheat flour

Brown rice
Wheat germ
Chicken
Peanut butter
Macaroni/spaghetti
Codfish
Soda crackers
Haddock
Peanuts
Lobster
Corned beef
Oatmeal
Sardines
Sausage
Dried lentils
Oysters
Scallops

Appendix 'F'

"Hidden Sugars" In Foods

Food Item	Size of Portion	Approx. Sugar content in teaspoonsful of granulated sugar
BEVERAGES		
Cola Drinks	1(6 oz. bottle or glass)	3 ½
Cordiails	1(3.75 oz. glass)	1 ½
Ginger Ale	6 oz.	5
Hi-Ball	1(6 oz. glass)	2 ½
Orange-Ade	1(8 oz. glass)	5
Root Beer	1(10 oz. bottle)	4 ½
Seven-Up	1(6 oz. bottle or glass)	3 ¾
Soda Pop	1(8 oz. bottle)	5
Sweet Cider	1cup	6
Whiskey Sour	1(3 oz. glass)	1 ½
CAKES & COOKIES		
Angel Food	1(4 oz. piece)	7
Apple Sauce Cake	1(4 oz. piece)	5 ½
Banana Cake1	(2 oz. piece)	2

Cheese Cake	1(4 oz. piece)	2
Chocolate Cake, Plain	1(4 oz. piece)	6
Chocolate Cake, Iced	1(4 oz. piece)	10
Coffee Cake	1(4 oz. piece)	4 ½
Cup Cake, Iced	1	6
Fruit Cake	1(4 oz. piece)	5
Jelly-Roll	1(2 oz. piece)	2 ½
Orange Cake	1(4 oz. piece)	4
Pound Cake	1(4 oz. piece)	5
Sponge Cake	1(4 oz. piece)	2
Strawberry Shortcake	1 serving	4
Brownies, unfrosted	1(¾ oz. Serving)	3
Chocolate Cookies	1	1 ½
Fig Newtons	1	5
Ginger Snaps	1	3
Macaroons	1	6
Nut Cookies	1	1 ½
Oatmeal Cookies	1	2
Sugar Cookies	1	1 ½
Chocolate Eclair	1	7
Cream Puff	1	2
Donut, Plain	1	3
Donut, Glazed	1	6
Snail	1(4 oz. piece)	4 ½

Appendix 'F'

"Hidden Sugars" In Foods. cont'd

Food ltem	Size of Portion	Approx. Sugar content in teaspoonsful of granulated sugar
CANDIES		
Average Chocolate Milk Bar		
(example: Hershey bar)	1 (1 ½ oz.)	2 ½
Chewing Gum	1 stick	½
Chocolate Cream	1 piece	2
Butterscotch Chew	1 piece	1
Chocolate Mints	1 piece	2
Fudge	1(1 oz. square)	4 ½
Gum Drop	1	2
Hard Candy	4 oz.	20
Lifesavers	1	⅓
Peanut Brittle	1 oz.	3 ½
CANNED FRUITS & JUICES		
Canned Apricots	4 halves & 1 Tbsp. syrup	3 ½
Canned Fruit Juice		
(swtnd)	½ cup	2
Canned Peaches	2 halves & 1 Tbsp. syrup	3 ½

Fruit Salad	½ cup	3 ½
Fruit Syrup	2 Tbsp.	2 ½
Stewed Fruits	½ cup	2

DAIRY PRODUCTS

Ice Cream	⅓ pint (3 ½ oz.)	3 ½
Ice Cream Bar	1	1 - 7
depending on size		
Ice Cream Cone	1	3 ½
Ice Cream Soda	1	5
Ice Cream Sundae 17		
Malted -Milk Shake	1(10 oz. glass)	5

JAMS & JELLIES

Apple Butter	1 tbsp.	1
Jelly	1 tbsp.	4 - 6
Orange Marmelade	1 tbsp.	4 - 6
Peach Butter	1 tbsp.	1
Strawberry Jam	1 tbsp.	4

DESSERTS, MISCELLANEOUS

Apple Cobbler	½ cup	3
Blueberry Cobbler	½ cup	3
Custard	½ cup	2
French Pastry	1(4 oz. piece)	5
Jello	½ cup	4 ½

Appendix 'F'

"Hidden Sugars" In Foods, cont'd.

"SUCROSE" CONTENT OF 24 LEADING CEREALS

Kelloggs Apple Jacks	%	52.04
Post Fruity Pebbles		48.51
Ralston Purina Cookie Crisp		45.45
Quaker King Vitamin		42.40
Post Super Sugar Crisp		42.16
Quaker Cap'n Crunch		39.09
'Kellogs Frosted Flakes		39.07
General Mills Trix		37.27
General Mills Golden Grahams		29.90
Kellogs Cracklin' Bran		27.50
Kelloggs Country Morning		21.85
Nabisco 100% Bran'		19.77
Kelloggs Frosted Mini Wheats		19.77
C. W. Post		18.20
Quaker 100% Natural		17.09
Kretschmer Sun Country Granola with almonds		16.82
Ralston Purina Bran Chex		14.25
Post Raisin Bran		12.97
Kelloggs 40% Bran Flakes		12.88
Kelloggs Raisin Bran		12.20

Kelloggs Rice Krispies	8.62
Wheaties	8.60
Kelloggs Corn Flakes	5.03
Cheerios	3.07

Appendix 'G'

United States Department of Agriculture list of the twelve most contaminated fruits and vegetables:

Celery
Apples
Bell peppers
Cherries
Grapes (imported)
Nectarines
Peaches
Pears
Potatoes
Red raspberries
Spinach
Strawberries

Contamination was measured AFTER the ftuits and vegetables had been washed! !

Appendix 'H'

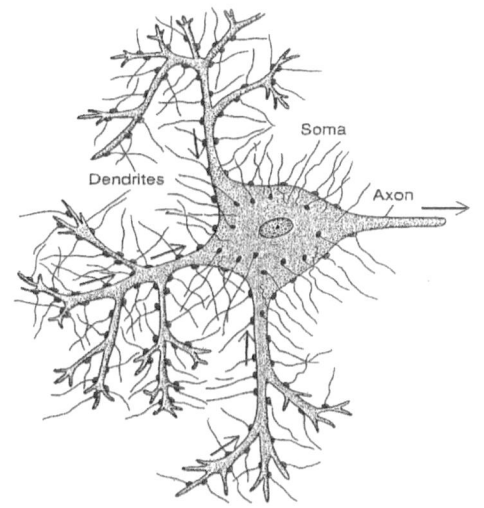

FIGURE "A"

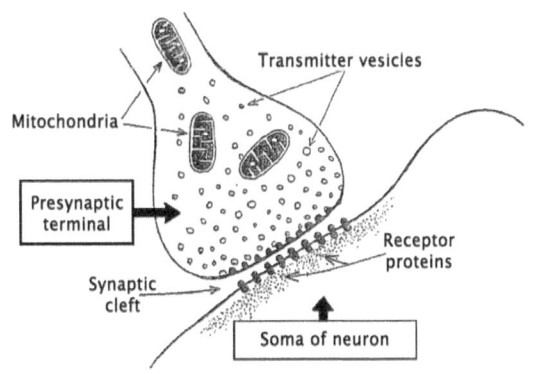

FIGURE "B"

Appendix 'I'

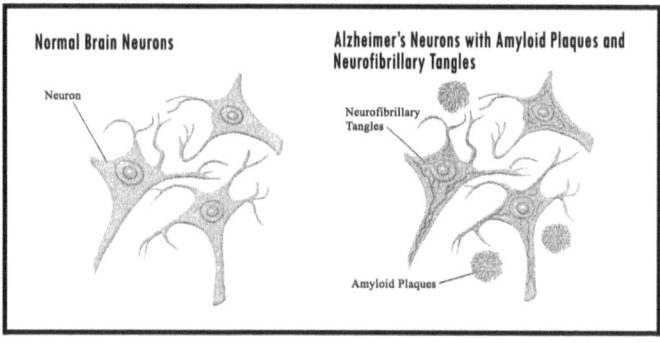

Normal Brain Neurons

Neuron

Alzheimer's Neurons with Amyloid Plaques and
Neurofibrillary Tangles

Neurofibrillary
Tangles

Amyloid Plaques